Opponent Process Theory

Justin W. Gibson • Brett A. Pearce
Robert C. Thomas
Steven D. Thurber

Opponent Process Theory

Neurophysiological Foundations and Clinical Applications

Springer

Justin W. Gibson
Louisiana State University Health Sciences Center
New Orleans, LA, USA

Brett A. Pearce
Louisiana State University Health Sciences Center
New Orleans, LA, USA

Robert C. Thomas
New York University School of Medicine
New York, NY, USA

Steven D. Thurber
Louisiana State University Health Sciences Center
New Orleans, LA, USA

ISBN 978-3-032-00089-7 ISBN 978-3-032-00090-3 (eBook)
https://doi.org/10.1007/978-3-032-00090-3

This Springer imprint is published by the registered company Springer Nature Switzerland AG
The registered company address is: Gewerbestrasse 11, 6330 Cham, Switzerland

Justin W. Gibson: I would like to dedicate my contribution contained in this work to my beloved grandmother, Mary Lou Hilts. She is the most selfless person I have ever known. Her whole life has been dedicated to helping for others, whether it was her family through being a loving mother and grandmother, giving children free books in her bookstore, or through church and civic service. Throughout my entire life, she has been a constant source of inspiration, love, and kindness and the greatest and most steadfast support I have ever had. She is truly an angel waiting for her wings.

Brett A. Pearce: I dedicate this to my parents, Bob and Julie Pearce, who have served as my therapists, confidants, emergency contacts, and occasional reality checkers for as long as I can remember. Your steady support and genuine care continue to shape the way I think and live. Also, to my nephew Zion Adams—thank you for reminding me that joy can be loud, messy, and wildly contagious

Robert C. Thomas: I dedicate my contributions in this work to my parents, Robert and Tama Thomas, and my brother, Michael Thomas, who have always been my biggest supporters. I also dedicate this to Dr. Annie Bowles-Welch, my first research mentor during my time as a fledging academic working toward my undergraduate neuroscience degree. Finally, I dedicate this to Trey DePhillips, without whom my world would be a much dimmer and duller place.

Steven D. Thurber: To my friend, colleague, critic, and esteemed daughter, Janean Thurber Yingling. You have encouraged and facilitated my ventures in research and publishing; you have provided wise counsel and candid evaluations; with gratitude and affection.

Preface

Years ago, I encountered an inmate in the California Prison system who was receiving emergency medical care for a major self-inflicted injury (major cut into her upper arm with a sharp object). Her explanation for what amounted to a protracted history of self-injuries was to the best of my recollection: "You know, it really hurts when I cut myself, but shortly thereafter I feel a wave of euphoria like nothing I experienced when I used opiates." As an early career psychologist, I at least realized the folly of reifying the phrase "euphoria follows self-induced pain" based on the self-report of a single incarcerated inmate. Nevertheless, her expression of a contrasting emotional aftereffect to pain prompted wonder as to whether such a phenomenon might exist. And the inmate's words describing an extreme hedonic contrast remained a memorable clinical experience for me.

Subsequently, I worked in a private hospital for the treatment of chemical usage disorders. One of my duties was to provide information to patients about the nature of addiction. As I combed the literature to acquaint myself with various explanatory models, I found the contributions of Richard Solomon (see Chap. 1). There was something that seemed vaguely familiar about their theorizing, viz., a pronounced emotional experience that in turn provokes an emotional contrast. But unlike the pain and affective upheaval of self-inflicted injuries, Solomon and Corbit's model began with a self-administered substance with attendant emotional elevation followed by an "opponent process," or negative affective condition. Moreover, this model explicitly proposed a definition of addiction as a shift from an initial motive to produce a positive emotional state to motivation pertaining to reducing the negative hedonic contrast. That is, when substance usage behavior is activated toward the goal of reducing an adverse opponent condition, addiction is the defining state of being (see more about opponent process theory and addiction in Chap. 3).

Many of the patients with whom I worked seemed to be perplexed by the mysterious "illness" of addiction. Although any mental health professional should view clinical experiences with a healthy dose of skepticism, it was my clinical impression that in the main, patients viewed the opponent process theory as valuable in fostering understanding of addiction. Many indicated that addiction had become a more denotatively exact, demystified term.

The notion of writing a book on opponent process theory was germinated in weekly informal interchanges among the four co-authors in the Psychiatry Department, Louisiana State University Health Sciences Center in New Orleans. I was the faculty member of the group, Drs. Pearse and Thomas were Psychiatry residents, and Gibson, a valued research associate in the department.

In part, we were meeting to identify shared interests that might be parlayed into a joint contribution to the Behavioral science/ Psychiatry literature. Of the several topics pondered, there was a converging interest in chemical usage disorders.

Over time, Opponent Process Theory (OPT) was broached as an explanatory model for chemical addiction, and the formulations of OPT heightened the collective epistemic curiosity of our group. As we further explored published data on OPT, we were enlightened and indeed surprised by studies outside the confines of chemical usage disorders, in fact across a diverse range, from forms of psychopathology to explanations of certain altruistic behaviors. For me, that stored memory of the inmate's pain infliction was revivified with research documenting instances of euphoric aftereffects of induced pain.

The OPT approach to addiction and its various extrapolations were compelling to our group to the extent that we organized our thinking and integrated the OPT data into a Psychiatry department poster presentation. This was followed by a book proposal, and we hope, a worthwhile literary product.

As authors, we contributed equally; hence, the decision to list authorship in alphabetical order. Nevertheless, we diversified in our OPT interests. Dr. Pearce was captivated by OPT and addiction; Gibson was especially curios about historical precursors and neurophysiology, while Dr. Thomas was intrigued by risk-taking and criminal behavior. I directed my attention to literature on pain, self-injury, food addiction, and therapeutic ramifications of OPT. We were all intrigued (and surprised) by extant research extending OPT to topics such as blood donation and facial afterimages.

In the course of reviewing relevant literature, we discovered that esoteric ideas about opposing forces were widespread. There were obvious religious traditions such as good in opposition to evil. There were also philosophical musings on polarities, and models of psychopathology like Freud's moral superego opposing the pleasure-seeking Id. There were abundant data on opposing homeostatic dynamics in physiology such as those involved in body temperature regulation, and even formulations and data at the quantum field level (e.g., matter versus antimatter). Then, and importantly, there were the unassailable, palpable facts about excitatory and inhibitory cells producing opponent color afterimages in vision research. These are just some of the noteworthy opponent process epochs (see elaboration in Chap. 1).

There is sufficient evidence to conjecture that thoughts about forces in opposition have been around for a long time in religious and philosophical ruminations that preceded the entry of opponent process notions into scientific discourse and hypothesis testing. Subsequent research findings and related consequential formulations of Solomon and others constitute essential elements of this book.

The phrase "Opponent Process Theory" or its acronym are used throughout our text. In science, the word "theory" is reserved for an evidence-based, substantiated explanation for natural phenomena. More than that, a theory provides predictions that can be verified or potentially refuted; it generates research. Additionally, a scientific theory is responsive to research findings and will be modified or possibly overturned as accumulating data dictate.

Specific to psychiatry and human services, a good theory should have practical ramifications, procedures for improving the human condition. Indeed, there are promising treatment approaches derived from OPT principles discussed in Chap. 8. In the aggregate, it is opined that the data presented in the text will justify attaching the appellation "theory" to opponent process.

New Orleans, LA, USA Steven D. Thurber

Acknowledgments

Faculty and Staff of Louisiana State University Health Sciences Center, New Orleans, Department of Psychiatry, Forensics Division: Dr. Rahn Bailey, Dr. Bing Simpson, Chikira Barker, Victoria Sacco, Margaret Heine, and Melissa Musacchia-Matory. Gratitude for the support and effort behind the scenes, without which this book would never have happened.

Drs. William Sheehan and William Meller of the Itasca Brain and Behavior Association and the University of Minnesota (Twin Cities) Medical School for reviews of the manuscript and valuable comments.

Contents

1 Historical Precursors

Beginning

Greetings! We would like to begin this intellectual journey with a type of experiment that will likely engender a sensory experience of an opponent process. It is our hope that this will transform the topic of this text from an abstract, esoteric idea into an authentic, palpable event, one that will be recalled throughout the following pages. Please, indulge us and follow these instructions:

1. Select a blank sheet of white paper.
2. Visually focus on the middle (white dot) of the flag shown in Image 1.1 for 30–60 s.
3. Shift gaze to the white sheet of paper.

In a few seconds, you should directly observe an opponent process in the visual system. The original green turns red in the after image. If this does not occur, please repeat the process.

We will return to the importance of the visual afterimage in historical context later in the chapter.

We have all experienced joy and happiness, gloom, and despair. Most often such emotions are directly related to the nature of an event or events and are appropriate to the circumstance. We also note that emotions in response to a particular situation often fail to reach the same level of intensity with repetition. Nevertheless, the

J. W. Gibson et al., *Opponent Process Theory*,
https://doi.org/10.1007/978-3-032-00090-3_1

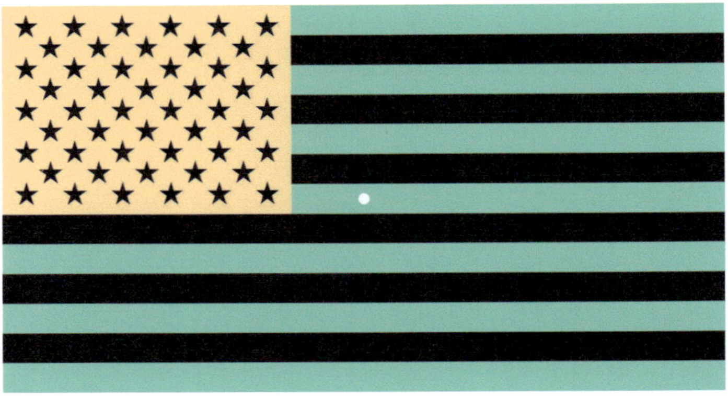

Image 1.1 Reverse colored American flag. (Usage Rights Granted by IStock)

general reliability and predictability of emotional experiences allow us to navigate effectively in our social and inanimate environments.

There is another dimension of emotional experience that exists and, like the strange realm of quantum mechanics in physics, follows laws that may be counterintuitive and escape personal awareness. It is termed "opponent process theory (OPT)," with dynamics we are beginning to comprehend and quantify, yielding data that may be important for understanding addictions, certain behavioral anomalies, and even altruistic activities. Such phenomena will be explored in this book.

We talk about and experience the ups and downs of existence. We look forward to the end of a workday with the anticipation that after a morning and afternoon of monotony and tedium, the emotional outlook will be better. We wonder about people who inexplicably seem to enjoy the tedium, the so-called "work-alcoholics." We hear about strange behaviors in others who inflict self-injuries; we read about or experience bipolar problems that can involve extreme fluctuations of emotions from elation to depression. Some of us have addictions to licit or illicit chemicals. All of these seemingly disparate phenomena may actually have a common element related to *opponent processes.* Moreover, and ironically, opponent processes associated with maladjustments, psychiatric disorders and addictions, actually stem from the body's natural adjustment and adaptation capacities gone awry.

Historical Antecedents of Opponent Process Theory

The concept of forces working in opposition to one another in order to create a balanced middle is as old as intellectual thought. This tendency continued through the Middle Ages, through the renaissance and enlightenment, and up to the modern age. Human beings tend to interpret reality as collections of competing forces, rather than benign phenomena.

Opposing Forces Across Cultural Mythology and in Antiquity

Opposite energies, aspects, and the balance (or lack thereof) have been part of the human mythos since before recorded history. These concepts are woven to the narratives told around the campfire and revered in shamanic spiritualism [1]. The masculine and feminine archetypes, how we each embody both aspects to varying degrees, and how these proportions influence our personality was understood as axiomatic by our early human ancestors [2]. These were linked to order and chaos by association with day and night, respectively. The sun deity was frequently depicted as masculine and representing order and the known while the moon deity usually represented feminine energy and was often associated with the unknown, mysterious, and chaos. That which emerged from the balance between these forces was believed to be the cycle of the natural world. Further, it represents the balance between the authoritative masculine and the nurturing feminine. It is, in fact, this balance between order and chaos, the known and unknown, predictable and unforeseen, which can be interpreted as the balance between stability and the need for novelty that exists in humans even to this day [3–5].

Some Specific Links to OPT in Religion, Philosophy, and Physics

The earliest historical contributions to human knowledge and reasoning included notions of contrasts and opposing forces. A sine qua non of vintage religious writings was the polemic of good versus evil. From Hinduism, for example, comes "Dharma," the personification of the righteous, "ought to" in morality in opposition to the unrighteous, "ought not" Adharma [6]. In Zoroastrianism, the corresponding polemical personages are "Ahura Mazda" and "Angra Mainyu," and in certain Abrahamic traditions such as Judaism and Christianity, the "good-evil" opposition is depicted by Yahweh versus Satan and Jesus versus the devil and other evil spirits. A more recent Christian denominational iteration accentuates the "importance of opposition in all things" [7–9] (Image 1.2).

In philosophy, Goethe was noted for his emphasis on opponent forces or polarities (e.g., characters in "Faust"), while Aristotle discussed the human condition related to being confronted by the

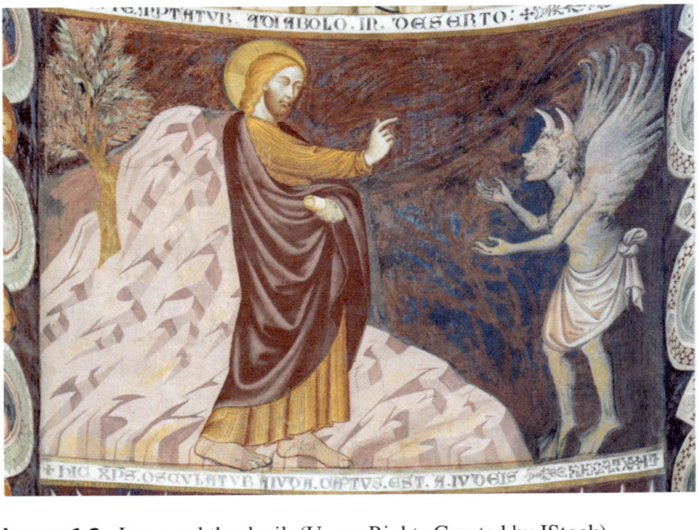

Image 1.2 Jesus and the devil. (Usage Rights Granted by IStock)

opposite extremes of excess and deficiency. He also proposed the "golden mean," pertaining to the notion of finding and adhering to the midpoint in reconciling extreme positions [10–12].

Finally, and obviously of profound significance, there are certain fundamental laws of physics, such as Dirac's confirmed notion of matter and antimatter, paired particles with the same mass but opposing electrical charges, as well as Bohn's opposing spin of entangled particles in quantum mechanics. Such conceptions suggest the importance of opposing forces as explanatory constructs in relation to the nature of physical reality [13, 14].

Resolution of Opposing Viewpoints and Contradictions in Philosophical Discourse

In what is termed "dialectic argumentation," exemplified by Plato's dialogues, there is a back-and-forth presentation of opposing ideas between interlocutors with the goal of some type of reconciliation or a balancing of contrasting positions. The German philosopher Hegel extended dialectics from polemical social interchanges to more abstract, epistemological considerations. In the Hegelian Dialectic process, one begins with a philosophical statement. This is the thesis. This is followed by a posited opposite of that statement, which is the antithesis. Through intellectual analysis, the two opposite concepts are combined into the synthesis. So here we see that two opposing concepts interact to form the balanced middle ground (similar to Aristotle's previously mentioned "golden mean") [15, 16].

The Zeitgeist in the Emergence of OPT

The zeitgeist of opposing forces, resolution and adaptation, were part of the cultural Milieu in which opponent process theory (OPT) originated.

Physiological Homeostasis

From micro to macro levels of analysis, biochemical, neurological, and behavioral processes function reciprocally to promote adjustment and adaptation. Maintaining an optimal body temperature (37 °C), for instance, pertains to a "biological thermostat" involving responsiveness to heat generated by internal organs in concert with extant external conditions. When needed, a complicated regulatory system is activated with a "sensor" of skin temperature, sensory information transmitted to the cerebral cortex and preoptic brain areas, resulting in sweating, if too warm, and shivering, if too cold. The hypothalamus, an important brain structure involved in hunger and thirst motivation as well as temperature regulation, triggers the biochemistry for body temperature homeostasis [17].

Useful Analogy

The old playground equipment termed "seesaw" or "teeter-totter" provides a simple, useful analogy or symbolic representation for homeostasis and later opponent process theory. Recall the seesaw has a long board with a pivot point; two children sit on either end, facing each other. Initially the board is balanced (Image 1.3).

As one child pushes up, the child on the other end of the teeter-totter goes down (Image 1.4), and the balance is disrupted, as illustrated below. Likewise, OPT pertains in part to disruptions in emotional states, similar to one end of the teeter-totter abruptly going up, and a compensatory opposite end undergoing a downward trajectory.

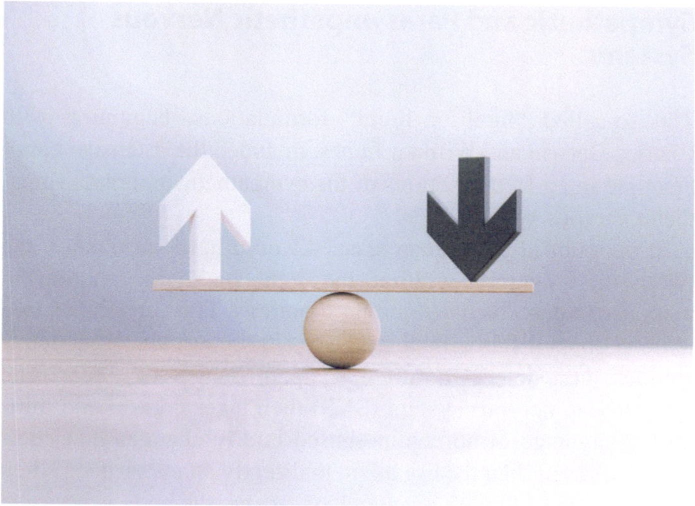

Image 1.3 Balanced opposing forces. (Usage Rights Granted by IStock)

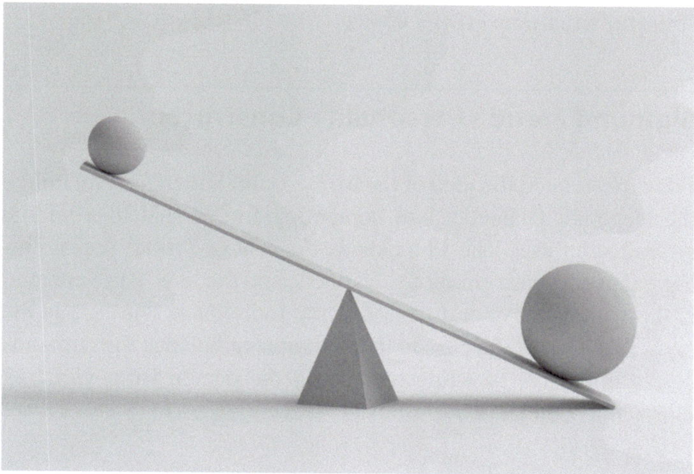

Image 1.4 Unbalanced opposing forces. (Usage Rights Granted by IStock)

Sympathetic and Parasympathetic Nervous Systems

The so-called "fight or flight" formulations, beginning with Charles Darwin and William James, included the ostensive opponent and integrated functions of the sympathetic and parasympathetic nervous systems.

It is doubtful the human species would have survived to the twenty-first century without the fight or flight reaction in response to perceived dangerous situations. The amygdalae, two almond-shaped subcortical structures in the left and right hemispheres, first detect stimuli that signal danger or threat. The sympathetic nervous system (SNS) then takes control and initiates a sequence of adrenaline-based bodily changes that energize and strengthen the organism to directly attack or flee. When the danger is dealt with via attack or escape, the body is returned to a more calm and subdued condition, via the parasympathetic nervous system (ANS). That is to say, the SNS and ANS have contrasting effects that may synergize into overall adaptation to stressful situations [18].

Sigmund Freud's Personality Constructs

Freud postulated the idea of the Id, Ego, and Superego. Not unlike the Hegelian Dialectic, two competing forces lead to a middle ground synthesis. The Id exists as the seat of primal urges, biological needs, base emotions, instincts, and the like. The Superego is the controlling moral center of the individual. The Ego is the conscious part of the person that attempts to balance the demands of the impulsive Id while preventing the person from violating moral and societal conventions [19].

Darwin's Theory and Adaptation

Charles Darwin's theory of evolution through natural selection is recognized as the very foundation for understanding and progress in the biological sciences. The notion that population traits are selected (i.e., lead to increased reproduction rates) based on progenitor adaptation to environmental challenges has influenced medicine and the behavioral sciences and was part of the scientific and intellectual climate in which OPT emerged [20].

Piaget's Theory

The typically developing child constructs working models of the outside world for understanding or *assimilating* information about that world. That world of reality for an infant may consist only of objects that impinge on the sensory organs. Thus, mother exists only when she can be seen, touched, heard, etc. So long as a particular model facilitates adequate navigation of one's social and physical environment, the formulation will continue to be employed. When new or more complicated challenges emerge, adaptation occurs through a modification or *accommodation* of an extant model or in the mental construction of a new model of reality. The notion that objects and people continue to exist albeit they currently cannot be seen or touched is an accommodation (change) that better fits the nature of reality and hence facilitates adaptation. When the child continues to use a model or mental schema even after it has outlasted its usefulness, there is assimilation with distortion, a form of cognitive maladaptation. That is, the child in effect forces information into the inadequate model and in so doing distorts that information. One can also *accommodate* or change models even though an existing model is working well. In both instances, the developing child is not in a state of adaptation, either assimilating with distortion or changing models prematurely. The dynamic forces are out of balance or in a state of disequilibrium.

The point is that *assimilation* and *accommodation* can oppose each other and be out of balance or they can equilibrate and synchronize. When the individual strikes a balance between assimilation and accommodation, *equilibration* or a reasonable degree of adaptation is extant [21].

Also, of note, is that following Piaget death, theoreticians have suggested a new, advanced stage in Piaget's theory of cognitive development, apparently influenced in part by the dialectics of Plato and Hegel. The proposal is that whereas earlier Piagetian stages involve progressive, reality-based cognitions for problem solving, the more advanced level is that of problem-finding. This refers to being attuned to, seeking out, and being epistemically curious about issues that may be opposing and contradictory and applying rationality for reconciliation and resolution [22]. Dialectic reasoning includes notions that two contradictory ideas can both have elements of truth, that "either-or" hypotheses for example (e.g., intelligence is determined either by genetics or environmental influences), have a potential resolution in an interaction hypothesis for investigation. Importantly, dialectical thinking pertains to understanding levels of complexity in phenomena and in one's own thought processes [23].

Return to Visual Afterimages

Perhaps the strongest single influence on the origin of Opponent Process theory was research on visual color afterimages. We hope you have now experienced this opponent process in our "experiment" in the beginning of the chapter with the green flag image repeated in Image 1.5. This is an opponent phenomenon that one can actually "see" in a very brief period. It is a directly observed opponent process in the visual system. The original green turns to the complimentary color red in the after image. Without going into physiological detail, one reason for this phenomenon is that green and red are opposing colors; there is no such thing as "greenish-reddish." The simple physiological explanation is that there are red cells and green cells (cones) in the retina, one of which is excitatory and the other inhibitory that connect to a gan-

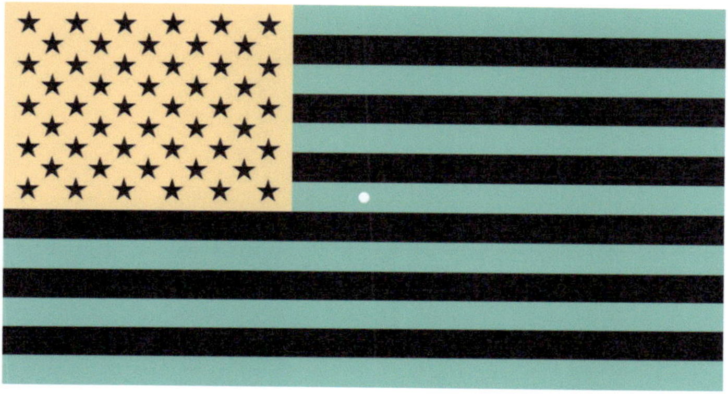

Image 1.5 Reverse colored American flag. (Usage Rights Granted by IStock)

glion cell the goes to the visual center of the brain. If the green cell excites, the perception will be green, while the red cell is simultaneously inhibitory. And, of course, the reverse occurs when the red input is excitatory [24].

Richard Solomon and Opponent Process Theory

In point of fact, the opponent visual afterimage and related theorizing of Hurvich and Hurvich [24] on explanatory neural processes may have constituted the major influence on psychologist Richard Solomon's subsequent expositions on oppositional emotional and behavioral dynamics.

Another antedating impact was Solomon's familiarity with the extreme emotional fluctuations of military parachutists making their first jumps during training [25]. Prior to the actual event, the parachutists were observed to show extreme signs of distress-irregular breathing, bulging eyes with dilated pupils, very stiff, stone-like postures, and facial expressions. In striking contrast, after a successful jump, the parachutists appeared a little stunned for a while and then began to interact joyously as if in a state of euphoria, eventually returning to a more balanced emotional condition.

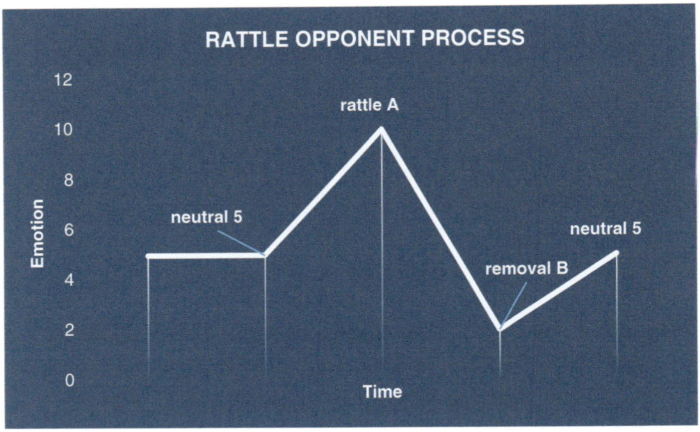

Fig. 1.1 Rattle opponent process. (Steven Thurber)

A simplified mainstream example of a negative opponent process is the infant who handles a rattle for the first time (Fig. 1.1). Initially the baby can be viewed as in a neutral emotional state of equilibrium. A bright colored rattle is presented to an infant who proceeds to grasp and shake the object; we observe a slight smile and other signs of mood elevation, as the child seems at least mildly entranced by the feel and sound of the object. Then the rattle is removed:

$$\text{Neutral state} \rightarrow \text{Rattle} \rightarrow \text{Happy expressions} \rightarrow \text{Rattle removed}$$

The infant then displays mood and behavior changes suggesting anger and sadness; this condition is emotionally opposite to the emotional elevation and is hedonically below the initial neutral condition. The baby, in effect, would have been better off emotionally had the rattle not been presented. Nevertheless, in a relatively brief period of time, the infant will likely return to the neutral pre-rattle condition.

$$\text{Neutral} \rightarrow \text{Mild distress, hedonic contrast} \rightarrow \text{Return to neutral state}$$

Most of us have probably experienced a type of "mild addiction" involving the ingestion of salted peanuts or small sugarcoated chocolate candies. It is often difficult to stop the ingestion. Once we do stop, there will be a craving to continue, but this B opponent process will be of relatively short duration. The noteworthy opponent process conditions result in a protracted B process.

It may be important to keep these exemplars (parachutes; rattles) in mind, along with the teeter-totter analogy, as we progress to more technical explanations:

A. The opponent process in color vision is a readily demonstrable opponent process that occurs in a matter of seconds (albeit very complicated in terms of visual and neurological explanations).
B. The example of baby and rattle illustrates a sequence from equilibrium to positive emotional change, countered by a hedonic contrast, and then a return to the neutral emotional condition. This is the basic model for an initial positive emotional state followed by an opposite affective condition.

Foundation Principles in Opponent Process Theory (OPT) [26–29]

An environmental event (e.g., chemical ingestion; parachute jumping; ingesting a favorite food) produces an emotional imbalance. Of particular relevance are intense, out of the ordinary, emotional experience. From the concept of homeostasis, the individual is in a state of disequilibrium and perhaps in a potentially maladaptive internal physiological condition.

In opponent process terminology, the initial emotion is the "primary condition," referred to as the "A state." It has a very rapid onset, but also a very rapid decline. It can be of high valence (ingesting an opiate) or more adverse in nature (electric shock), but it may be extreme to the extent of a pronounced disruption of one's optimal adaptation level. The "A" emotion is then countered by a "hedonic contrast" that opposes the A state and functions in part to reduce or neutralize the primary affective reaction. Unlike the A state however, the hedonic contrast or "B" state is slow in its decay. And in emotional homeostasis, the individual actually experiences a condition in contrast to the initial A state. A simple example, likely experienced by most persons in modern society, would be eating salted peanuts or potato chips. The initial ingestion may produce an elevated pleasurable emotion that eventually "wears off." This is followed by a negative condition conceptualized as a type of craving that is only reduced by ingesting another handful of the salted snacks.

In a drug-induced example, the primary A state caused by opiate ingestion is rather ephemeral and is "pulled down" or neutralized by the emerging hedonic contrast or B state. Let's say that a first-time drug-using individual decides one time is enough; he or she never uses again. The aversive counter effect or B state will then undergo its slow decay and that will be the end of it. On the other hand, imagine this naïve drug-user ingests a second drug while the B state is still in the process of slow dissipation. What then, are the ramifications? First, the active B condition will yield a type of force on the second A state such that it does not reach the same level of elevation. Second, the B condition now starts above zero and hence "builds" from a higher existing intensity level, in effect from the wave of the initial B state that has not decayed completely. If the individual continues producing the A state while the B state is active and building, then addiction will be forthcoming. In opponent process theory, addiction is defined as a shift in motivation. In the beginning, motivation is geared toward the anticipated pleasure of the primary condition (A state). Addiction occurs when as the result of frequent chemical usage, the motivation is shifted to the ingestion of alcohol or another drug in order to reduce the aversive B state (anxiety, depression, cravings, and other withdrawal symptoms). An important corollary is that the highly elevated, pleasurable A condition is never again achieved, at least not to the same ecstatic degree (this is usually termed "tolerance").

Of course, the same opponent dynamics obtain if the initial A condition is adverse (e.g., extreme physical exercise). In such instances, there may be motivation toward maintaining or increasing the strength of the positive hedonic B contrast.

In the chapters to follow, we will review a wide range of phenomena, beginning with neurophysiological underpinnings of

Opponent Process Theory, and proceeding to opponent processes that underpin certain maladaptive behaviors and more commonplace activities. A later chapter will address therapeutic modalities that conflate with OPT principles.

References

1. Shipley TE. Opponent-processes, stress, and attributions: some implications for shamanism and the initiation of healing relationships. Psychother Theory Res Pract Train. 1988;25(4):593–603. Available from: https://doi.org/10.1037/h0085386.
2. Greenfield B. The archetypal masculine: its manifestation in myth, and its significance for women. J Anal Psychol. 1983;28(1):33–50. Available from: https://doi.org/10.1111/j.1465-5922.1983.00033.x.
3. Halsberghe GH. Sol Invictus Elagabal. In: The cult of Sol Invictus. Brill; 1972. p. 45–107. Available from: https://doi.org/10.1163/9789004296251_005.
4. Díaz H, Maureira F, Cohen E, Córdova F, Palominos F, Otárola J, et al. Individual differences in the order/chaos balance of the brain self-organization. Ann Data Sci. 2015;2(4):421–38. Available from: https://doi.org/10.1007/s40745-015-0051-y.
5. Hussenot A, Missonier S. Encompassing stability and novelty in organization studies: an events-based approach. Organ Stud. 2016;37(4):523–46. Available from: https://doi.org/10.1177/0170840615604497.
6. Selwyn T. Adharma. Contrib Indian Sociol. 1981;15(1–2):381–401. Available from: https://doi.org/10.1177/006996678101500120.
7. Smarandache F. The dynamic interplay of opposites in zoroastrianism. J Fuzzy Ext Appl. 2024;5:1–15.
8. Russell JB. The prince of darkness. Cornell University Press; 2016.
9. Smith J. 1830 Book of Mormon. A Marvelous Work and A Wonder; 2007.
10. Cardinal CH. Polarity in Goethe's Faust. Publ Mod Lang Assoc Am. 1949;64(3):445–61. Available from: https://doi.org/10.2307/459745.
11. von Goethe JW. Faust, Faust II. New Haven: Yale University Press; 1998.
12. Aristotle. Nicomachean ethics. Cambridge: Cambridge University Press; 2000.
13. Rafelski J, Birrell J, Steinmetz A, Yang CT. A short survey of matter-antimatter evolution in the primordial universe. Universe. 2023;9(7):309. Available from: https://doi.org/10.3390/universe9070309.
14. Horodecki R, Horodecki P, Horodecki M, Horodecki K. Quantum entanglement. Rev Mod Phys. 2009;81(2):865–942. Available from: https://doi.org/10.1103/revmodphys.81.865.

15. Maybee J. Hegel's dialectics. In: Zalta E, editor. Stanford encyclopedia of philosophy. Stanford University; 2020.
16. Kraut R. Plato. In: Zalta E, editor. Stanford encyclopedia of philosophy. Stanford University; 2022.
17. Koyama Y, Hosomi S, Yoshiya K. Editorial: Body temperature homeostasis: the biological thermostat. Front Neurosci. 2024;18:1527270. Available from: https://doi.org/10.3389/fnins.2024.1527270.
18. Ondicova K, Mravec B. Multilevel interactions between the sympathetic and parasympathetic nervous systems: a minireview. Endocr Regul. 2010;44(2):69–75. Available from: https://doi.org/10.4149/endo_2010_02_69.
19. Freud S. An outline of psychoanalysis. Oxford: W. W. Norton; 1963.
20. Darwin C. The origin of species. London: HarperCollins Publishers; 1963.
21. Phillips J. The origins of intellect. W. H. Freeman; 1975. Available from: https://doi.org/ISBN10:071670580X/ISBN13:9780716705802.
22. Ho DYF. Dialectical thinking: neither eastern nor western. Am Psychol. 2000;55(9):1064–5. Available from: https://doi.org/10.1037/0003-066x.55.9.1064.
23. Arlin PK. Cognitive development in adulthood: a fifth stage? Dev Psychol. 1975;11(5):602–6. Available from: https://doi.org/10.1037/0012-1649.11.5.602.
24. Hurvich-Jameson D, Hurvich LM. Opponent-colors theory and physiological mechanisms. In: The visual system: neurophysiology and psychophysics. Springer; 1961. p. 152–63. Available from: https://doi.org/10.1007/978-3-662-22221-8_19.
25. Fenz WD, Epstein S. Gradients of physiological arousal in parachutists as a function of an approaching jump. Psychosom Med. 1967;29(1):33–51. Available from: https://doi.org/10.1097/00006842-196701000-00005.
26. Solomon RL, Corbit JD. An opponent-process theory of motivation: I. Temporal dynamics of affect. Psychol Rev. 1974;81(2):119–45. Available from: https://doi.org/10.1037/h0036128.
27. Solomon RL. The opponent-process theory of acquired motivation: the costs of pleasure and the benefits of pain. Am Psychol. 1980;35(8):691–712. Available from: https://doi.org/10.1037/0003-066x.35.8.691.
28. Solomon R, Corbit J. An opponent-process theory of motivation. Am Econ Rev. 1978;68:12–24.
29. Solomon RL. Further implications of opponent-process theory. Behav Brain Sci. 1978;1(3):459. Available from: https://doi.org/10.1017/s0140525x0007607x.

Neurophysiological Underpinnings

2

Some Elementary Facts About the Brain and Opponent Process Theory

The notion that opponent processes exist at a behavioral level may be unassailable. The intriguing mystery is what may occur in brain circuitry and biochemistry to produce the equilibrating impact of opponent dynamics. Thankfully, there are some excellent hypotheses that are generating research and provide foundational data. We will begin with a basic discussion of the brain and its neurotransmitters and modulators and then proceed to a more technical presentation.

Imagine looking Inside the brain; almost exactly in the middle is the Ventral Tegmental Area or VTA. A component substructure of the VTA is the Nucleus Accumbens (sometimes termed the "pleasure center"). A close neighbor of the VTS is the Hypothalamus (often called the "motivation center"). These are key structures in Opponent Process Theory and will be discussed and illustrated throughout our text in some detail.

Neurotransmitters

The brain is composed of cells (about 100 billion) called neurons. These cells are interconnected and indeed messages in the brain

J. W. Gibson et al., *Opponent Process Theory*,
https://doi.org/10.1007/978-3-032-00090-3_2

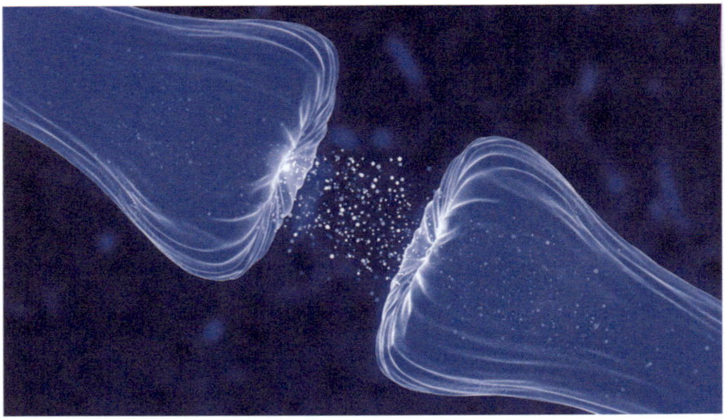

Image 2.1 Synapse. (Usage Rights Granted by IStock)

(i.e., thinking) require electrical impulses to traverse across typically a very large number of neurons. However, these brain cells do not actually touch each other. As illustrated in Image 2.1, there is a space between neurons (called the synaptic gap) that must be "bridged" in order for the brain to "work." The neurotransmitters (there are many specific to brain circuity) are chemicals that fill the gap and allow excitation or inhibition of neuronal pathways. The neuron "sending" the electrical message via a particular neurotransmitter connects with other neurons that function as appropriate receptors for that neurotransmitter. One neurotransmitter important in opponent process theory is "dopamine," related to elation and euphoria. Another neurotransmitter of import is the "corticotropin-releasing factor" (also a hormone) critical to the anti-reward or stress system, much more to come on these neurotransmitters.

Neuromodulators

Unlike neurotransmitters, a neuromodulator does not directly excite or inhibit neurons that receive an electrical message. Rather, they alter or regulate how neurons respond to neurotransmitters.

Hormones, neurotransmitters, and neuromodulators are conceptually similar in that they all relate to regulation of the body; the difference is whether that regulation occurs via brain cells (neurotransmitters and neuromodulators) or in the cells and tissues outside the brain (hormones).

Neuromodulators then modify the effects of neurotransmitters (e.g., making receptor neurons more difficult to excite). Central to opponent process is a group of neuromodulators called "opioid peptides," the most relevant of these for our purposes is called "dynorphin." This will be important in our later discussion of pain and opponent processes.

Opponent Neurophysiological Dynamics

The body maintains a state of physiological homeostasis. Temperature, blood pressure, and other physical states are maintained by achieving balance between competing forces. Neurologically, this is also the case. The resting state of neurological systems in the body is not the absence of process, but rather a balance of excitatory and inhibitory processes. One can observe layers of balance, from the macro/system level down to the cellular level. These processes stabilize thought, emotion, and behavior. This is particularly evident when examining the neurological roots of approach/avoidant behavior and appetitive/aversive stimuli. The phenomenon is observable in the brains of humans, other primates, as well as rodents, suggesting that this is a biological standard across mammal species. These are the stimuli and behaviors with which this chapter will be primarily (though not exclusively) concerned, involving competing excitatory and inhibitory stimuli as well as opposing behavioral impulses and expressions.

Background

First, we would like to provide a brief overview of some concepts that are relevant to this chapter as well as chapters to come. There are some brain-related terms that are known and familiar to most readers. There are also concepts such as approach/avoidance, appetitive/aversive, and neuronal polarity that will be explored. It is also necessary for the reader to have some understanding of the function of certain brain structures such as the nucleus accumbens (NAc), pregenual cingulate cortex, (pACC), pontine central grey area, and paraventricular thalamus. Further, it is crucial that the reader be aware of the function of certain neurotransmitters, including Gamma-Aminobutyric Acid (GABA), acetylcholine (ACH), and glutamate.

Approach/Avoidance

Decision making is based on an approach/avoidance paradigm. Whenever a choice is made, the opponent processes of approach and avoidance are in competition with one another. Imagine an individual making a large purchase such as an automobile or home. There is a drive towards the reward of acquiring the product. However, there is likely going to be some trepidation regarding the forfeiture of money that the purchase requires. The individual is experiencing competing, opposite impulses [1].

More About Neurotransmitters

Of the two excitatory neurotransmitters discussed in this chapter, perhaps glutamate is primary. It operates on receptors such as N-methyl-D-aspartate (NMDA) [2]. Acetylcholine is the other important excitatory neurotransmitter. Though most often discussed in regard to nerve impulses between nerves and muscle tissue, it also plays an important role in many brain structures [3]. GABA is primarily an inhibitory neurotransmitter of which glutamate is a precursor, though under select circumstances it can act in an excitatory manner. GABA is important due to its function in regulating neuronal impulses [4].

Brain Structures

The NAc is part of a brain network involved in emotions and cognition regarding appetitive and aversive stimuli, primarily through the effects of dopamine transmission [5]. Image 2.2 shows many structures involved in this process. The pregenual anterior cingulate cortex (pACC) is a complex brain structure involved in many different processes, including emotions (such as anxiety and fear), cognition, and inhibition of action, to highlight a few. It has also been shown to be associated with social cognition [6]. The pontine central grey contained in the pons, a structure found in the brain stem. It is associated with approach/avoidance behavior [7]. The ventral palladium is a structure which has long been connected to motor function. More recently, it has also been implicated as a reward structure associated with motivation [8]. The thalamus operates as a relay station to rout signals from one brain structure to another. The paraventricular thalamus (PVT) connects the reward circuit pathways from the prefrontal cortex to the limbic system [9]. It also receives projections from the hypothalamus. There is evidence that the PVT is involved with numerous

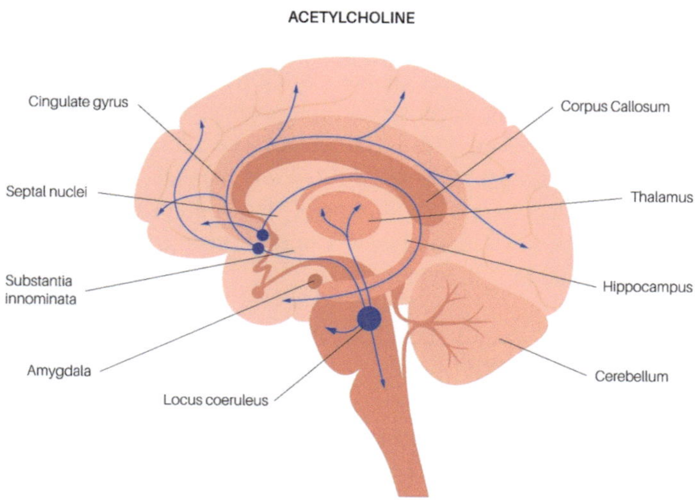

Image 2.2 Brain structures. (Usage Rights Granted by IStock)

components of behaviors related to substance use due to its association with reward- and goal-directed behavior [10]. The pregenual cingulate cortex is a brain structure involved in decision making, specifically in the analysis of cost and benefit [11]. The striatum is a structure with which many other brain regions are associated. It plays a crucial role in learning, stimuli association and reinforcement, and many other behavioral functions. While there is significant functional segregation in the striatum, there may also exist interaction among signals from many brain structures [12].

Neuronal Polarity

The functionality of the neuron itself is dependent on opposing forces. The propagation of action potential is the result of both concentration and charge gradients which exist between the cellular interior and the extracellular environment. The neuron resting state is at an internal charge of −70 mV. The extracellular environment is positively charged. Homeostatic balance within the cell is maintained by passive ion channels allowing for the gradual passage of sodium, potassium, and chloride ions as well as the sodium/potassium pump, which hydrolyzes an ATP molecule to move two sodium ions out while transferring one potassium ion in. This balance is interrupted when the nerve receives an impulse. If the impulse is sufficient to depolarize the neuron to −55 mV. This causes voltage-gated ion channels to open, and the neuron depolarizes. At this point, the sodium ion channels close and the potassium channels open, causing the neuron to repolarize, and in fact, hyperpolarize [13].

Ligands and OPT

Three primary ligand molecules influence the way we think, feel, perceive, and act. Image 2.3 shows the cellular structures upon which these ligands operate. These are glutamate and acetylcho-

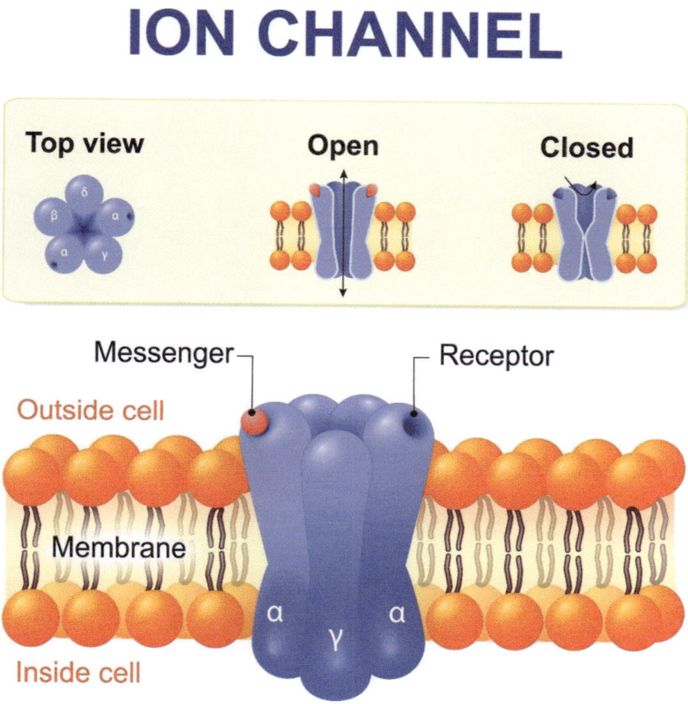

Image 2.3 Ligand gated channel. (Usage Rights Granted by IStock)

line, shown in Image 2.4 (excitatory) and GABA, shown in Image 2.5 (inhibitory). These neurotransmitters operate in opposition to one another, creating a push/pull effect. Many studies have shown that there is no simplistic explanation for the interactions between these neurotransmitters. For example, it has been found that GABA can exert inhibitory influence when released in certain brain structures but is also co-released alongside Ach when other brain regions are stimulated. This co-release is of particular interest, as it could function to reduce interference from certain neurons that would inhibit the stimulus response. However, it could possibly involve a process akin to a b-state as described by OPT [14].

It was found, in rats, that there is an interplay between Ach and GABA. Glutamate agonists such as NMDA caused an increase in

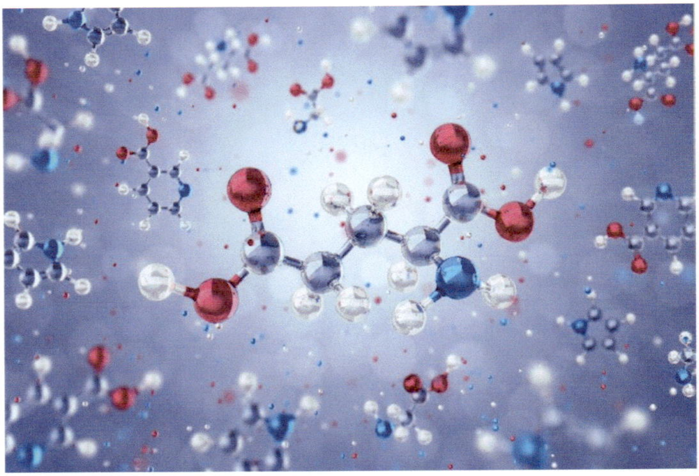

Image 2.4 Glutamate. (Usage Rights Granted by IStock)

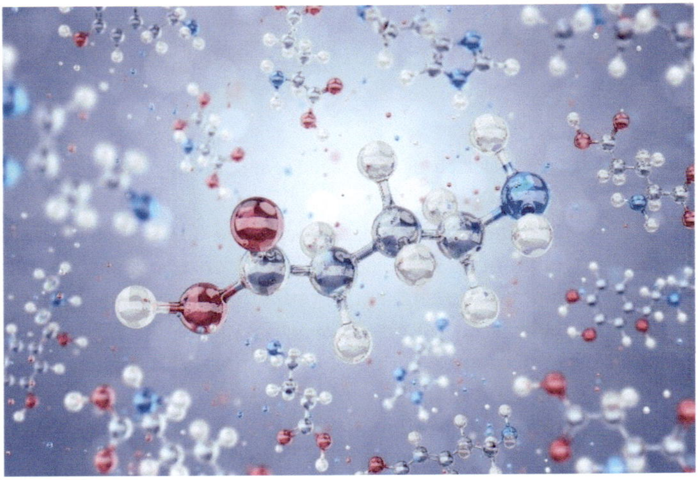

Image 2.5 GABA. (Usage Rights Granted by IStock)

levels of extracellular dopamine as well as GABA. However, there was a temporal delay in the increase of GABA. One may recall that, in opponent process, there is a temporal delay between the onset of the A state and the B state. It is also postulated that glutamate may have a dual role, both excitatory and inhibitory. This is consistent with the concept put forward in this chapter that the neurochemistry and electrochemical activity of the brain is one of balance between opposing excitatory and inhibitory ligands [15].

Striatal Neurons (Excitatory Neurons and Inhibitory Interneurons)

There is one finding regarding low-threshold spiking (LTS) interneurons in the striatum, shown in Image 2.6, that is of interest to this topic of discussion. Nicotinic receptor activation seems to elicit competing excitatory and inhibitory responses. When stimulated with tonic Ach, there is a direct excitatory effect. But there is also an increase in tonic GABA. Further, muscarinic activity inhibits LTS interneurons while also causing a reduction in GABA inputs. We see here yet another example of competing forces at the neurobiological level [16].

Brain Structures, Competing Forces, and OPT

The nucleus accumbens, highlighted in orange in Image 2.7, presents an interesting example of a structure in which opponent process is particularly evident. This is the primary reward pathway for the brain. As such, it is a crucial region for approach/avoidant behavior as well as conditioning. It receives projections from, and projects to a number of other structures. Glutamatergic, cholinergic, and GABAergic neurons all play a role in the functions of the

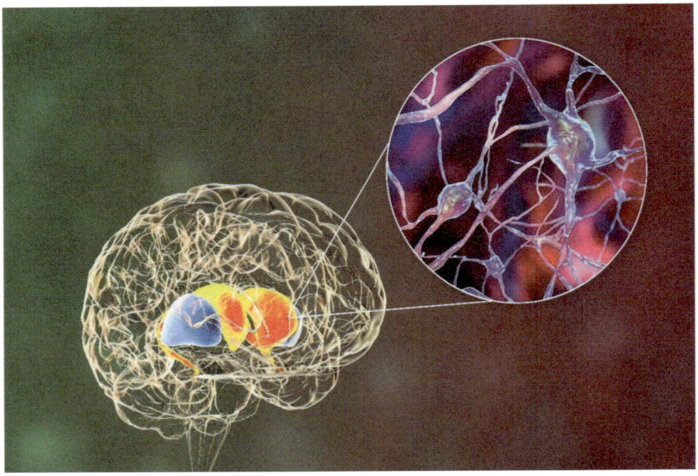

Image 2.6 Dorsal striatum. (Usage Rights Granted by IStock)

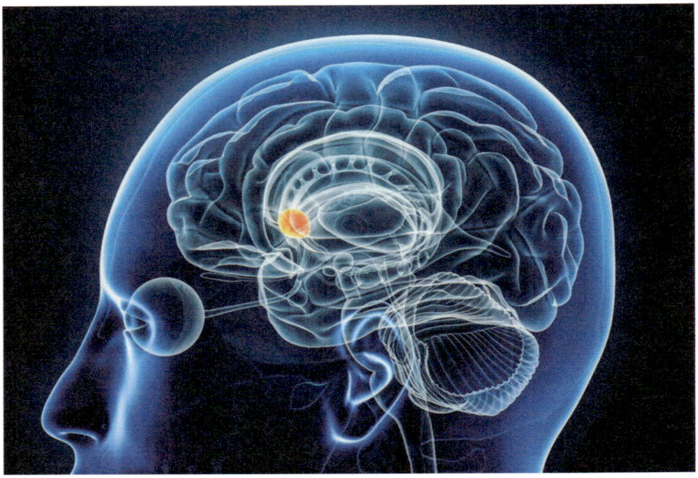

Image 2.7 Nucleus accumbens. (Usage Rights Granted by IStock)

NAc. In some instances, glutamatergic and cholinergic projections into the structure evoke an inhibitory effect, whereas GABAergic neurons elicit excitatory neuronal activity within the NAc. This indicates that both the projections and the neurons within the structure are operating as opposing processes, striking a balance between excitatory and inhibitory impulses which is perturbed when an event occurs eliciting either appetitive or aversive behavior [17].

GABA and Glutamate neurons in the ventral palladium display parallel projections within this structure and may act in opposing roles. These project to dopamine neurons throughout the nucleus accumbens. In fact, according to one study, bulk dopamine neuron activation increases even though these neurons can result in opposing effects. Dopamine release in the ventromedial NAc shell is aversive, whereas the same in the dorsomedial shell is rewarding. Further, this study found that some of the same cells are activated for both appetitive and aversive stimuli. This could indicate that this state creates an opposing balance with these cells providing a moderating impulse working opposite of the observed behavioral impulse [17].

In the pontine central gray area of the brain, GABAergic and glutamatergic neurons have been shown to affect valence-specific approach/avoidance behaviors. GABAergic neurons are associated with approach behavior, and glutamatergic neurons are associated with avoidance behaviors. Functionally, these cell groups operate in opposition to one another and initially create a neutral state. The addition of stimuli associated with either appetitive or aversive stimulus perturbs this neutral equilibrium [7].

It has been shown that, in the primate pregenual cingulate cortex, two groups of neurons operate to create opponent processes, eliciting either emotionally positive or emotionally negative behaviors in macaque primates. These processes play a role in approach/avoidance decisions and actions and evince a balance between approach and avoidance neurons operating in opposition to one another [11].

On a broader level, competing forces of excitation and inhibition are extant between more holistic brain regions and systems. Executive inhibitory control functions of the prefrontal cortex in relation to impulsive excitation and certain limbic functions is an exemplar (see Ref. [18]).

Conclusion

The neurochemistry and functions of the brain involve a balance of competing forces. This can be seen at the level of the individual neuron and up through the communication between complete brain structures. What we see in the brain is a complex dance of excitation and inhibition. Some neural systems activate in order to elicit action, some activate to exert inhibitory control over brain structures. This is particularly evident when examining how appetitive and aversive stimuli evoke approach/avoidant behaviors. These behaviors pertain to a balance between opposing forces of excitation and inhibition. This balance provides the neurochemical and physiological basis for the opponent process model.

References

1. McNally GP. Motivational competition and the paraventricular thalamus. Neurosci Biobehav Rev. 2021;125:193–207. Available from: https://doi.org/10.1016/j.neubiorev.2021.02.021.
2. Meldrum BS. Glutamate as a neurotransmitter in the brain: review of physiology and pathology. J Nutr. 2000;130(4):1007S–15S. Available from: https://doi.org/10.1093/jn/130.4.1007s.
3. Sam C, Bordoni B. Physiology, acetylcholine. In: StatPearls. Treasure Island: StatPearls Publishing; 2023.
4. Watanabe M, Maemura K, Kanbara K, Tamayama T, Hayasaki H. GABA and GABA receptors in the central nervous system and other organs. Int Rev Cytol. 2002;213:1–47. Available from: https://doi.org/10.1016/s0074-7696(02)13011-7.
5. Floresco SB. The nucleus accumbens: an interface between cognition, emotion, and action. Annu Rev Psychol. 2015;66(1):25–52. Available from: https://doi.org/10.1146/annurev-psych-010213-115159.
6. Palomero-Gallagher N, Hoffstaedter F, Mohlberg H, Eickhoff SB, Amunts K, Zilles K. Human pregenual anterior cingulate cortex: structural, functional, and connectional heterogeneity. Cereb Cortex. 2019;29(6):2552–74. Available from: https://doi.org/10.1093/cercor/bhy124.

7. Xiao C, Wei J, Zhang G, Tao C, Huang JJ, Shen L, et al. Glutamatergic and GABAergic neurons in pontine central gray mediate opposing valence-specific behaviors through a global network. Neuron. 2023;111(9):1486–1503.e7. Available from: https://doi.org/10.1016/j.neuron.2023.02.012.
8. Smith KS, Tindell AJ, Aldridge JW, Berridge KC. Ventral pallidum roles in reward and motivation. Behav Brain Res. 2009;196(2):155–67. Available from: https://doi.org/10.1016/j.bbr.2008.09.038.
9. Otis JM, Zhu M, Namboodiri VMK, Cook CA, Kosyk O, Matan AM, et al. Paraventricular thalamus projection neurons integrate cortical and hypothalamic signals for cue-reward processing. Neuron. 2019;103(3):423–431.e4. Available from: https://doi.org/10.1016/j.neuron.2019.05.018.
10. Zhou K, Zhu Y. The paraventricular thalamic nucleus: a key hub of neural circuits underlying drug addiction. Pharmacol Res. 2019;142:70–6. Available from: https://doi.org/10.1016/j.phrs.2019.02.014.
11. Amemori K, Graybiel AM. Localized microstimulation of primate pregenual cingulate cortex induces negative decision-making. Nat Neurosci. 2012;15(5):776–85. Available from: https://doi.org/10.1038/nn.3088.
12. Rolls E. Neurophysiology and cognitive functions of the striatum. Rev Neurol. 1994;150:648–60.
13. Tams N. Action potential: a tutorial study guide. Nicoladie Tam, Ph.D.; 2015.
14. Pepeu G, Blandina P. The acetylcholine, GABA, glutamate triangle in the rat forebrain. J Physiol Paris. 1998;92(5–6):351–5. Available from: https://doi.org/10.1016/s0928-4257(99)80004-7.
15. Hernández L, Segovia G, Mora F. Effects of activation of NMDA and AMPA glutamate receptors on the extracellular concentrations of dopamine, acetylcholine, and GABA in striatum of the awake rat: a microdialysis study. Neurochem Res. 2003;28:1819–27.
16. Elghaba R, Vautrelle N, Bracci E. Mutual control of cholinergic and low-threshold spike interneurons in the striatum. Front Cell Neurosci. 2016;10:111. Available from: https://doi.org/10.3389/fncel.2016.00111.
17. Faget L, Oriol L, Lee W-C, Zell V, Sargent C, Flores A, et al. Ventral pallidum GABA and glutamate neurons drive approach and avoidance through distinct modulation of VTA cell types. Nat Commun. 2024;15(1):4233. Available from: https://doi.org/10.1038/s41467-024-48340-y.
18. Otero T, Barker L. The frontal lobes and executive functioning. In: Goldstein S, Naglieri J, editors. Handbook of executive functioning. New York: Springer; 2014.

Substance Usage 3

Theoretical and Neurobiological Foundations

Opponent-Process Theory Overview

Solomon and Corbit originally proposed OPT as a general model of motivation and emotion, later applied to drug use and addiction [1]. The core concept is that a positive or pleasurable drug effect (A-process) is inherently followed by an opposing negative effect (B-process) as the brain strives for equilibrium. Early in drug use, the pleasurable A-state (e.g., euphoria, relaxation) dominates and the B-state is minimal. With repeated use, however, the B-process grows stronger and longer, while the A-process weakens. The initial drug "high" becomes shorter-lived, whereas the subsequent "low" (dysphoria, anxiety, craving) deepens and lasts longer [2]. This progressive intensification of the opponent B-state underlies tolerance (diminished drug effect) and withdrawal (pronounced negative symptoms when the drug wears off). Eventually, the user's motivational focus flips: instead of taking the substance to feel good, they take it primarily to avoid feeling bad. At this stage, drug use is sustained more by negative reinforcement (relief of discomfort) than positive reinforcement. This flip in motivation (the hallmark "dark side" of addiction) means each use only briefly alleviates an ever-worsening baseline state [3].

J. W. Gibson et al., *Opponent Process Theory*,
https://doi.org/10.1007/978-3-032-00090-3_3

Temporal Dynamics and Allostasis

As addiction develops, the timing and balance of the A- and B-processes change. Initially, the positive A-process dominates with only a delayed, small B-process. With continued use, the B-process onset becomes faster and its magnitude larger, eventually overshadowing the A-process. This progression has been framed in terms of allostasis or a gradual shifting of the brain's reward set-point to a new pathological equilibrium. Repeated drug exposure lowers the baseline ability to experience pleasure (a chronic reward deficit) and elevates baseline stress and dysphoria (a chronic stress surplus). Koob and colleagues describe addiction as a cycle wherein each intoxication temporarily restores normal mood but also drives the baseline mood further into negative territory [4]. In other words, the brain's efforts to maintain stability in the presence of drugs result in an "anti-reward" adaptation: the person's normal state becomes subnormal unless the drug is present. This could help explain why people escalate use and struggle with abstinence. This is because, when not using they are left in a protracted negative state that the drug temporarily relieves via negative reinforcement [4].

Neurobiological Mechanisms of Addiction

At the neural level, OPT corresponds to well-documented changes in brain circuitry during addiction. The primary A-process involves activation of the brain's reward pathways, notably the mesolimbic dopamine system (ventral tegmental area projecting to nucleus accumbens) along with other neurotransmitters (opioid peptides, endocannabinoids, GABA) that mediate the drug's acute positive effects. The opponent B-process is driven by counter-adaptations in these and related circuits [5]. With repeated drug use, within-system adaptations dampen the original reward signal (e.g., reduced dopamine release and receptor sensitivity in the nucleus accumbens, contributing to tolerance), while between-system adaptations recruit stress and aversive circuits that oppose the drug's effects. A key player is the dynorphin–kappa opioid system: chronic drug exposure increases the neuropeptide dynorphin, which activates kappa-opioid receptors that inhibit dopamine neurons. This puts a brake on reward circuitry and induces dysphoria and anxiety; elevated dynorphin during withdrawal produces profound anhedonia (inability to feel pleasure) unless the drug is used [6]. In parallel, the stress neurotransmitter corticotropin-releasing factor (CRF) becomes overactive in the extended amygdala (e.g., central amygdala and bed nucleus of the stria terminalis). High CRF during withdrawal causes intense anxiety, irritability, and sensitivity to stressors [7]. Thus, as addiction progresses, the brain's reward function is blunted while its stress systems are hyperactivated. The individual not only derives little pleasure from normally enjoyable activities but also experiences excessive discomfort and stress even at baseline. Notably, these opponent-process responses can be triggered by drug-associated cues or stressors even before actual withdrawal. For example, encountering a context linked to prior drug use or experiencing a stressor can evoke a mini-withdrawal state (craving, low mood, tension) via conditioned activation of these anti-reward circuits, contributing to persistent relapse vulnerability [7]. Chronic drug use also disrupts glutamate signaling between the prefrontal cortex (PFC) and the accumbens. Normally, PFC glutamatergic input helps regulate decision-making and inhibit impulsive actions, but in addiction this top-down control is weakened while drug-seeking habits are strengthened. The result is impaired impulse control and compulsive drug-seeking. Even if the individual wants to quit, the capacity of the PFC to override drug urges is compromised [8]. There is also evidence that chronic drug exposure engages neuroimmune and inflammatory processes in the brain, further altering neural circuits and contributing to mood and cognitive deficits, although these changes can vary by substance [9].

Individual Differences

Genetic and environmental factors influence how rapidly and intensely the opponent-process mechanism kicks in. For example, certain genetic profiles (affecting dopamine or stress pathways) or life experiences like chronic stress can predispose an individual to a stronger and more persistent B-process, whereas others with more resilient neurobiology may experience milder opponent effects [10]. Such differences may explain why only some drug users progress to severe addiction despite exposure.

In summary, repeated cycles of intoxication and withdrawal trigger neuroadaptive changes including decreased dopamine function, increased dynorphin and CRF activity, and other allostatic adjustments that create a persistent reward deficit and stress surplus in the addicted brain. Voluntary, pleasure-driven drug use evolves into compulsive, relief-driven use. Even after the individual stops taking the drug, residual opponent-process changes (an overactive stress system, weakened reward response, and conditioned cues that elicit craving) may linger for months or years, contributing to a high risk of relapse [11]. With this foundation in place, we can examine how these opponent-process dynamics manifest with specific categories of substances and how each drug's unique pharmacology interacts with the same fundamental A/B-process mechanism of addiction.

Substance-Specific Opponent-Process Mechanisms

Opioids: From Euphoria to Hyperkatifeia

Opioids (e.g., heroin, morphine, oxycodone) provide a classic demonstration of OPT. A-process (acute reward): Opioids bind to mu-opioid receptors, triggering a surge of dopamine in the nucleus accumbens and the release of endogenous opioids. This produces intense euphoria, pain relief, anxiolysis, and sedation. B-process (withdrawal dysphoria): With repeated opioid use, the body and brain mount opponent adaptations. Mu-opioid receptors become desensitized (phosphorylated and internalized), so the same dose releases less dopamine and yields less pleasure over time (tolerance). Simultaneously, opposing neurochemical systems are upregulated. Dynorphin levels rise in the nucleus accumbens, and by activating kappa-opioid receptors, they inhibit dopamine release, leading to dysphoria and anhedonia during withdrawal [6]. Likewise, stress neurotransmitters such as CRF are released in excess in the extended amygdala, eliciting intense anxiety and emotional distress [7]. The result is a severe negative state during withdrawal that Koob has termed "hyperkatifeia" which has been described as an extreme dysphoric stress state beyond normal homeostasis [2]. In practical terms, a dependent opioid user feels profoundly unwell without the drug: wracked by flu-like physical symptoms (aches, nausea, sweating) and emotionally on edge, unable to derive pleasure from normally enjoyable activities. Taking opioids again provides only temporary relief from this misery (negative reinforcement), but once the drug wears off, the agony returns. Research also shows that the lateral habenula, a region signaling negative reward, becomes hyperactive during opioid withdrawal and inhibits dopamine neurons, contributing to the extreme dysphoria [12, 13].

Overall, the opponent-process in opioid addiction is dramatic: over time the individual comes to need the opioid just to feel momentarily "normal," representing a complete reversal of the drug's original motivation (from seeking euphoria to avoiding dysphoria). Clinically, opioid withdrawal includes severe muscle and bone pain, gastrointestinal distress, gooseflesh, insomnia, intense anxiety, and overwhelming dysphoria. Symptoms can begin within hours of the last dose in a dependent person, reflecting how rapidly the opponent-process kicks in. Because this withdrawal syndrome is so aversive, users often relapse early or continue dosing just to avoid it. Recognizing the opioid opponent-process has informed treatment: maintenance therapies like methadone or buprenorphine occupy mu-opioid receptors to prevent the full swing into withdrawal, and experimental treatments targeting the kappa-opioid or CRF systems aim to blunt the intense “dark side” state to aid in recovery.

Psychostimulants: Crash, Anhedonia, and Stress-Primed Relapse

Psychostimulants (e.g., cocaine, methamphetamine) also evoke opponent-process dynamics, although stimulant withdrawal is largely psychological rather than overtly physical. A-process (acute reward): Stimulants sharply increase monoamine neurotransmitters, especially dopamine. Cocaine blocks dopamine reuptake (simultaneously elevating serotonin and norepinephrine), while amphetamines not only block reuptake but also trigger excess dopamine release. The result is a surge of dopamine in reward pathways, producing intense euphoria and alertness [14]. Stimulants also acutely increase glutamate release in reward-related regions, strengthening drug-related memories and associations. B-process (crash and adaptation): With repeated stimulant use, opposing processes build up. The brain reacts to chronic dopamine surges by downregulating the dopamine system: D_2 dopamine receptors become less available and dopamine synthesis/release decreases. Imaging studies in addicted individuals show reduced D_2 receptor levels and blunted dopamine release in the striatum compared to non-users [14]. As a result, the capacity to experience reward without the drug is greatly diminished. After a stimulant binge, users typically undergo a “crash” marked by extreme fatigue, low mood, and anhedonia. This crash can persist for days or even weeks as the brain’s reward circuitry is depleted and unresponsive. Normal activities that once brought pleasure no longer do, and only taking the stimulant can restore dopamine function toward baseline. Over time, stimulant abusers may develop a lasting depressive-like state. Chronic stimulant use also impairs prefrontal cortical function, weakening the “brakes” on drug-seeking behavior [8].

Stimulant withdrawal is primarily emotional but can be severe. In the aftermath of a binge, individuals often experience profound dysphoria, irritability, anxiety, and intense craving. The stress system is highly engaged: CRF levels rise in the amygdala during stimulant withdrawal (similar to opioids), creating hypersensitivity to stress. Blocking CRF_1 receptors in animal models attenuates stress-induced relapse to cocaine seeking, indicating that withdrawal-related stress is a key driver of craving and relapse [7]. Clinically, many stimulant users report that stress or negative emotions are major triggers for craving. Through the OPT lens, after repeated binges, the brain's baseline emotional state shifts to one dominated by dysphoria and stress, so any added stressor feels magnified and provokes a strong urge to use the drug as an escape.

Environmental cues associated with stimulant use can also trigger a conditioned opponent reaction. This can lead to a surge of craving accompanied by a dip in mood or spike in anxiety. These cues activate the anti-reward circuitry even in the absence of the drug, and with weakened prefrontal control [8], the person remains highly susceptible to relapse when encountering such triggers.

Alcohol: Tolerance, Allostasis, and Emotional Withdrawal

Alcohol (ethanol) addiction exemplifies opponent-process mechanisms involving both intense physical withdrawal and a significant emotional/stress component. Alcohol has broad actions in the brain, acutely producing euphoria, sociability, and anxiolysis (reduced anxiety); at higher doses, it causes sedation and motor impairment, and at extreme doses unconsciousness. Neurochemically, ethanol enhances $GABA_A$ receptor activity (increasing inhibition) and inhibits NMDA-type glutamate receptors (decreasing excitation). This overall suppression of neural activity leads to relaxation and mood elevation in the short term. Dopamine release in the nucleus accumbens is also increased by alcohol (though less directly than by stimulants), contributing to its rewarding effects [8].

With heavy chronic drinking, the brain counteracts alcohol's persistent depressant effects by dialing down inhibition and ramping up excitation. It does so by reducing the sensitivity of $GABA_A$ receptors and increasing the function of NMDA glutamate receptors, effectively "re-balancing" neural activity in the presence of alcohol. If alcohol is suddenly removed, this balance is lost: excess glutamate and inadequate GABA produce a state of hyperexcitability. This is the physiological basis of alcohol withdrawal syndrome. Symptoms include tremors, anxiety, insomnia, elevated heart rate, and blood pressure and in severe cases seizures or delirium tremens. The opponent-process overshoot, in part due to neural firing rebounding without alcohol's calming influence, makes alcohol withdrawal potentially life-threatening. In OPT terms, the B-process for alcohol is an extreme rebound in brain excitability [9].

Chronic alcohol use also causes a reward deficit and stress excess. Long-term drinkers often have reduced dopamine transmission in reward pathways, contributing to anhedonia and depression during sobriety. Moreover, alcohol withdrawal strongly activates stress pathways: CRF is released in the amygdala during withdrawal, producing intense anxiety and malaise. Administering CRF antagonists to dependent animals can relieve some withdrawal symptoms, underscoring CRF's role in alcohol's opponent process [7]. Alcohol dependence is also associated with an overactive hypothalamic–pituitary–adrenal (HPA) stress axis: even outside acute withdrawal, dependent individuals typically exhibit elevated stress hormones and an exaggerated stress response, and they commonly feel tense or on edge when not drinking.

Over time, additional neuroadaptations accumulate in alcoholism: sleep and mood-regulating systems become disrupted, and neuroimmune activity in the brain is heightened. These changes further contribute to the allostatic shift, or the brain's normal set-point for mood and arousal becomes pathologically altered such that alcohol is required to feel "normal" [9]. Thus, someone with severe alcohol dependence is essentially in a state of minor withdrawal whenever they are not drinking. They may experience persistent anxiety, irritability, and insomnia for weeks into abstinence. This prolonged opponent-process often precipitates craving: stress or negative emotions strongly trigger the urge to drink because the brain "remembers" that alcohol will alleviate the discomfort. Environmental cues (like being in a bar or reaching one's usual drinking time) can likewise induce craving by evoking the expectation of relief and the memory of how bad sobriety feels.

Future Directions in OPT Research

Individual variability in opponent processes: A key question is why some people develop much stronger opponent-process effects than others. The standard OPT framework does not explicitly include genetic, developmental, or psychosocial moderators. Recent research is examining how factors like genotype (e.g., variants in dopamine or opioid receptors) or pre-existing psychiatric traits influence the relative strength of the A- vs. B-process. For example, genetic differences in dopamine or stress systems and co-occurring mood or anxiety disorders may lead to an exaggerated B-process and a faster shift to relief-driven use [10]. Future computational models aim to incorporate such person-specific variables to predict who is most at risk for rapid opponent-process escalation.

Persistent Vulnerability After Abstinence

Even after prolonged abstinence, latent opponent-process adaptations can resurface. A recovering addict may experience a sudden wave of dysphoria and craving when exposed to a severe stressor or drug-associated cue, almost as if in withdrawal again. Drug-related cues become conditioned stimuli that automatically trigger elements of the B-state (negative mood, craving). Therapies aimed at disrupting these learned associations (e.g., during memory reconsolidation) are being explored. Clarifying the neural basis of this persistent vulnerability which sometimes viewed as a "scar" of addiction is considered vital to improving relapse prevention and reinforces the concept of addiction as a disease of pathological learning and memory [15].

Integration with Other Addiction Theories

Other models emphasize additional facets of addiction that complement OPT. For example, incentive sensitization theory posits that repeated drug use hyper-sensitizes "wanting" (craving) even as "liking" (euphoria) diminishes, so drug cues become powerful triggers for craving [16]. Likewise, habit formation models suggest that drug-seeking shifts from a conscious, goal-directed action to an automatic habit governed by stimulus-response loops in the dorsal striatum [17]. These perspectives intersect with OPT: the opponent-process creates a chronic negative drive state, while sensitized cues and ingrained habits channel the person toward drug use as the solution.

New therapeutic targets and strategies: Insights into opponent-process mechanisms highlight potential treatment approaches. For instance, because CRF plays a central role in the B-state, CRF_1 receptor antagonists have been trialed to mitigate withdrawal and prevent stress-induced relapse [7]. Similarly, the dynorphin–kappa opioid system has emerged as a target: blocking kappa-opioid receptors could relieve the dysphoric, anhedonic "dark side." Some experimental compounds (including certain buprenorphine metabolites that act as KOR antagonists) are being studied to see if they can shorten or lessen the withdrawal-related negative state [2]. Repairing glutamate disruptions is another angle: agents like N-acetylcysteine (NAC) and acamprosate aim to restore prefrontal control and reduce pathological cue-triggered craving by normalizing glutamate levels. These have shown promise in reducing cue-induced craving in some studies, consistent with reversing aspects of opponent-process-driven plasticity in the PFC–accumbens pathway. Beyond medications, brain stimulation approaches (e.g., transcranial magnetic stimulation or deep brain stimulation) are also being explored to reset opponent-process circuits by strengthening executive control or dampening overactive stress circuitry, thereby easing the negative emotional drive behind relapse.

Summary and Conclusion

Opponent-Process Theory offers a powerful framework for understanding why substance use, initially motivated by pleasure, often transitions into compulsive use motivated by the relief of distress. Across drug classes and beyond we see the same fundamental pattern, an acute positive drug effect (A-process) recruits an opposing negative effect (B-process) that grows with repeated exposure and eventually comes to dominate the user's emotional state. Psychologically, OPT captures the shift from positive reinforcement (using to feel good) to negative reinforcement (using to avoid feeling bad) that typifies advanced addiction. Neurobiologically, it maps this shift to concrete changes: downregulation of reward pathways (e.g., reduced dopamine signaling) and upregulation of stress/anti-reward pathways (e.g., increased dynorphin and CRF activity). In short, the brain's attempt to maintain homeostasis in the face of drugs leads to a new pathological equilibrium centered on a deficit of reward and an excess of stress.

By the time addiction is firmly established, the individual is fighting not just the drug's effects but also their own powerful opponent-process adaptations. The persistent "dark side" state, which is marked by anhedonia and chronic stress, can last long into abstinence and is a major driver of relapse. This reframes addiction as more than a series of impulsive choices; it is a chronic, adaptive disorder of the brain's reward and stress systems. Appreciating this has practical importance: it helps explain why willpower or short-term detox alone is often insufficient for recovery. Unless the opponent-process (withdrawal distress, protracted dysphoria, and cue-induced craving) is addressed, the person remains in an internal state that strongly pushes them back to drug use. Effective treatment therefore must work to restore balance by means of managing withdrawal symptoms, reducing stress, and helping the brain slowly recalibrate to a normal state. This may involve medications for detoxification and maintenance, behavioral therapies to cope with stress and triggers, and providing alternative rewards (exercise, social connection, etc.) to rebuild the ability to experience pleasure without drugs.

OPT is supported by extensive evidence, from tolerance and withdrawal phenomena to neuroimaging findings of altered neurocircuitry in addiction [18]. However, addiction also involves factors beyond OPT's scope such as craving can increase even as pleasure declines, and habitual drug-seeking can persist without strong craving or withdrawal. Thus, OPT is often integrated with other models such as incentive sensitization (pathological "wanting") and habit learning (automaticity of drug use). Notably, Baker et al. have reformulated addiction as an affective processing model centered on negative reinforcement, paralleling OPT's core tenet [19].

In conclusion, opponent-process theory remains a central organizing principle for understanding addiction. It reminds us that every euphoric high comes at the cost of an opposing low, and with chronic use, this "dark side" can eventually take over. Recognizing the opponent-process element of addiction fosters a more compassionate view of why people struggling with addiction find it so difficult to quit: they are often trapped not by the pursuit of pleasure, but by the avoidance of pain. It also directs scientific and clinical attention toward alleviating the negative emotional state of addiction, not just blocking the drug's initial effects. As research progresses, the details of OPT will continue to be refined, but its enduring insight is that in addiction, the brain's own counter-regulatory mechanisms become the enemy within and that taming this opponent is key to breaking the cycle and achieving recovery.

References

1. Solomon RL, Corbit JD. An opponent-process theory of motivation: I. Temporal dynamics of affect. Psychol Rev. 1974;81(2):119–45.
2. Koob GF. Neurobiology of opioid addiction: opponent process, hyperkatifeia, and negative reinforcement. Biol Psychiatry. 2020;87(1):44–53.
3. Koob GF, Le Moal M. Addiction and the brain antireward system. Annu Rev Psychol. 2008;59:29–53.

4. Ahmed SH, Koob GF. Transition to drug addiction: a negative reinforcement model based on an allostatic decrease in reward function. Psychopharmacology. 2005;180(3):473–90.
5. Koob GF, Volkow ND. Neurocircuitry of addiction. Neuropsychopharmacology. 2010;35(1):217–38.
6. Wee S, Koob GF. The role of the dynorphin–kappa opioid system in the reinforcing effects of drugs of abuse. Psychopharmacology. 2010;210(2):121–35.
7. George O, Le Moal M, Koob GF. Allostasis and addiction: role of the dopamine and corticotropin-releasing factor systems. Physiol Behav. 2012;106(1):58–64.
8. Kalivas PW, Volkow ND. The neural basis of addiction: a pathology of motivation and choice. Am J Psychiatry. 2005;162(8):1403–13.
9. Crews FT, Vetreno RP. Neuroimmune basis of alcoholic brain damage. Int Rev Neurobiol. 2014;118:315–57.
10. Sinha R. Chronic stress, drug use, and vulnerability to addiction. Ann N Y Acad Sci. 2008;1141:105–30.
11. Koob GF, Schulkin J. Addiction and stress: an allostatic view. Neurosci Biobehav Rev. 2019;106:245–62.
12. Matsumoto M, Hikosaka O. Lateral habenula as a source of negative reward signals in dopamine neurons. Nature. 2007;447(7148):1111–5.
13. Stamatakis AM, Stuber GD. Activation of lateral habenula inputs to the ventral midbrain promotes behavioral avoidance. Nat Neurosci. 2012;15(8):1105–7.
14. Volkow ND, Fowler JS, Wang GJ. The addicted human brain: insights from imaging studies. J Clin Invest. 2003;111(10):1444–51.
15. Hyman SE. Addiction: a disease of learning and memory. Am J Psychiatry. 2005;162(8):1414–22.
16. Robinson TE, Berridge KC. The incentive sensitization theory of addiction: some current issues. Philos Trans R Soc Lond Ser B Biol Sci. 2008;363(1507):3137–46.
17. Everitt BJ, Robbins TW. Drug addiction: updating actions to habits to compulsions ten years on. Annu Rev Psychol. 2016;67:23–50.
18. Volkow ND, Koob GF, McLellan AT. Neurobiologic advances from the brain disease model of addiction. N Engl J Med. 2016;374(4):363–71.
19. Baker TB, Piper ME, McCarthy DE, Majeskie MR, Fiore MC. Addiction motivation reformulated: an affective processing model of negative reinforcement. Psychol Rev. 2004;111(1):33–51.

Commonplace Behaviors with Opponent Process Foundations

4

Exercise, Opponent Process and Dual-Mode Theory

Brief Digression

This chapter includes two formulations that are putative "theories." We digress briefly to address the question of what constitutes a theory. If we have two "theories" that purport to explain the same data, in this case the positive emotional change following a period of physical exercise, then we cannot say they both have attained theoretical equivalence. A theory represents the apex is science, a formulation that adequately explains and integrates extant data, generates hypotheses for further investigation, and at least temporarily occupies ascendance in these domains. If another formulation challenges an established theory, its claim to superiority in relation the above criteria would of have to be demonstrated.

Dual-Mode

In the area of exercise and emotional change, the first explanatory "model" is termed "Dual-Mode" [1]. The initial mode pertains to the physiological underpinnings of emotionality. Mode number

J. W. Gibson et al., *Opponent Process Theory*,
https://doi.org/10.1007/978-3-032-00090-3_4

two is cognitive; the specific nature or type of one's emotion experience relates to thinking and rational evaluation. In part, or perhaps in the main, the dual-mode model was inspired by the work of Schachter and Singer [2], which we will now elaborate.

Schachter, Singer Two-Factor Theory

Volunteer participants at the University of Minnesota were informed (actually misinformed) that the purpose of the study was to investigate various visual skills and how such skills might be related to vitamins, especially the vitamin compound labeled "suproxin." In reality, the vitamin compound of interest was the genuine hormone/neurotransmitter "epinephrine" that mimics the discharge of the sympathetic nervous system in the flight/fight reaction. The impact of this discharge results in increased systolic blood pressure, heart rate, and respiration, with peripheral blood decreases, together with increases in blood sugar and lactic acid concentrations.

Research participants received two forms of "suproxin," either genuine epinephrine in the experimental group or a placebo. The latter was a saline solution.

Another experimental manipulation involved the information given participants regarding side effects of the "suproxin." Some participants received an appropriate explanation of the physiological sequalae of epinephrine (e.g., heart pounding, shaking of hands); others were given non-appropriate expectations of side effects such as itching or numbing of feet. And importantly, a third group simply remained uninformed.

The final level of deception in this research was the use of confederates to model behaviors congruent with either anger or euphoria. For example, an individual would be joined by a confederate who complained about being involved and displayed other signs of agitation. In a separate instance, a participant was accompanied by a confederate who states the visual skills assessments made him feel like a child again while evincing happy child-like behaviors such as building paper airplanes.

Subsequent data indicated that in the absence of an adequate explanation for the experienced physiological effects of suproxin, participants receiving epinephrine sought an explanation in the cognitive appraisal social available social cues, viz., the actions and demeanor of their assigned confederate. The outcome was either euphoria or anger consistent with the statements and affective expressions of the confederate.

The confirmed hypotheses in the Schachter/Singer study resulted in a two-factor model of emotion: (1) physiological arousal and (2) cognitive appraisal. That is to say, the physiological concomitants are presumed to be general across emotional conditions, and in the absence of explicit understanding of the cause of the physiological changes, the specific emotional condition experienced is dependent on a cognitive evaluation of available environmental cues. The Dual-Mode model (or theory) for the affective experiences of exercise appears to be a straightforward application of the Schachter/Singer approach: Arousal and Appraisal. However, the source of the arousal, exercise, is directly available, unambiguous, and somewhat inconsistent with the Schachter/Singer formulations.

The Role of Cognition in Emotion

In opponent process theory, higher order thinking is largely discounted; this may be a deficiency in current theory postulates. The a and b processes are mainly subcortical, albeit as we will discuss in the chapter on food addiction and eating disorders, higher level cognitions pertaining to thoughts about body image and fears of gaining weight may have an adverse effect on opponent processes and homeostatic adjustments. In the Dual-Mode approach, the cognitions include attributions (assignment of causation), self-efficacy (e.g., confidence on one's ability to attain a particular goal), interpersonal processing, and monitoring of interoceptive stimuli influence affective experiences. Moreover, cognitive factors may be more important than physiological arousal at lower levels of exercise intensity [1, 3].

Exercise and Opponent Process Theory

Opponent Process Reminders of Import in Exercise

In theory, the "A" process responds immediately in proportion to the strength of the presenting stimuli (complex stimuli pertaining to physical exercise) and returns to the initial baseline level when exercise concludes. The "B" process responds more slowly but proportional to "A" intensity.

Although there is a paucity of studies on the topic of exercise, extant research suggests an important explanatory role for opponent process theory that interacts with levels of exercise intensity. The criterion for extreme exercise exertion is termed the "lactate threshold or LC," defined as the lactate level beyond a capacity for adequate removal during exercise.

In the study by Markowitz and Arent [3], for example, the "A" process of exercise anxiety only occurred with intensity levels 5% above LC. It is noteworthy, however, that a positive "B" process was not identified after exertion terminated. In fact, tension and anxiety actually increased, post-exertion. It may be that the Dual-Mode cognitive component may provide a better understanding of emotionality and exercise. Nevertheless, extreme physical exercise may be unique in opponent process application given the post-exertion recovery time required for dissipation of accelerated physiological processes such as oxygen consumption. Markowitz and Arent [3] reported that after a more prolonged recovery period, the positive "B" state would likely emerge. Earlier Data from Gaesser and Brooks [4] support such a conclusion.

Lochbaum and Bixby [5] compared physically unfit persons to individuals considered physically fit on acute periods of aerobic exercise. Consistent with opponent process theory, all participants were found to have more negative affect during exercise, and a more positive "rebound" affect after exertion. In addition, more physically fit persons experienced elevated degrees of positive affect compared to other participants. Further, higher intensity exercise elicited less positive emotionality in contrast to low intensity exertion. Nevertheless, findings of similar levels of post-exercise affect, regardless of fitness and exercise intensity, are challenging to opponent process theory.

In addition to the intersection of opponent process theory with exercise intensity, there is at least partial support for OP theory relative to increased positive affect and reduced anxiety levels during and following acute activity on an exercise bicycle. However, this corroboration of OP predictions was robust only for individuals with a history of active exercise practice; non-active participants were found to evince reduced positive and negative affect during exercise and only a slight affective increase post exercise [6].

Work: Job Satisfaction and Opponent Process Theory

Perhaps you have heard the platitude, "work wouldn't be work unless you'd rather be doing something else," or the contrasting term "workalcoholic." These juxtaposing notions from common parlance may reflect that work, by definition, is aversive; anyone who states they love to work is either lying or being self-deceptive. Yet there are those who engage excessively in physical and mental "work" and may express an enjoyment in work-related activities. The "enjoyment" may relate to the secondary pleasurable aftereffect; they are addicted to the opponent process.

Of course, opponent process theory provides a very simple explanation. Yes, work of any type is aversive, creating negative emotionality. But the more one engages in work the stronger the opponent hedonic aftereffect. We work to enjoy the hedonic contrast when work terminates. However, it is not quite that simple when applied to emotional satisfaction relative to more complicated interacting variables on-the-job.

Job satisfaction is multifaceted. As presented by Landy [7], job satisfaction may pertain to an employment challenge that produces an adverse hedonic condition that may persist until the challenge is met; then the primary process is gradually replaced by the contrasting pleasurable aftereffect. Depending on the nature of one's employment, there may be repeated aversive challenges that vary in primary process strength and attendant inhibitory pleasurable consequences.

Adding to the complexity of job satisfaction is the fact that work is not play (duh). Play involves engagement in activity in which there is not external incentive (e.g., money) for such engagement. How might a financial incentive relate to work and job satisfaction? There are other extrinsic factors that contribute to job satisfaction that have implications for opponent process dynamics such as the quality of peer interactions and promotions. In contrast to work challenges, such factors may produce negative aftereffects.

Currently, job satisfaction and opponent process theory have several reasonable hypotheses that have yet to be rigorously investigated. For instance, will an employment reward such as promotion result in mood elevation that due to an opponent process attenuate over time to baseline? Will an employee report negative affect with an assigned task before meeting the designated objective? (see Refs. [7, 8]).

Repeated Blood Donations and Opponent Process Theory

Blood donation may be a pure form of altruistic behavior; it involves a degree of personal sacrifice, at least mild pain and discomfort, typically without monitory incentive and void of a hint of some type of reciprocity. What could motivate such behavior on the part of presumed self-centered homo sapiens?

Piliavin et al. [9] investigated the hypothesis that the initial adverse emotional experience of blood donation, perhaps engendered by a sense of social responsibility, results in an aversive experience that over repeated instances is replaced by a positive hedonic contrast. What appears as selfless behavior, and indeed an initial donation may accurately described as such, repeated, habitual blood donations may become a form of philosophical hedonism; That is, personal pleasure may be the "moral" principle guiding the individual's conduct.

Regardless of the philosophical considerations of repeated blood donations, opponent process theory may provide a plausible pleasure-centered explanation for voluntary behaviors that in the beginning are unpleasant.

The opponent process-related investigation followed a familiar model. With multiple instances of blood donation, an initial primary condition (A state) bill become less intense, the effect of the opposing B process. The A condition will continue to be reduced in intensity, approaching the baseline level. Correspondingly, the opposing B state becomes longer lasting in contrast to the first few instances of blood donation.

Piliavin et al. [9] obtained self-report data from 116 individuals prior to their initial blood donations. Subsequently the group attained a median of six donations and a mean of over eight. The participants provided pretest ratings (four-point scale) across adjectives denoting emotionality. Adjectives best denoting the A state were *uptight, dubious, fearful, skeptical, jittery, regretful, suspicious, angry, defiant and rebellious*. Corresponding B state adjectives included, *carefree, playful, kindly, witty, warmhearted, vigorous, and relaxed*. The B condition adjectives were administered post-donation. In addition, two 7-point ratings were gathered pertaining to the participant's emotionality during the puncture phase and about 3 min after puncture.

Consistent with theoretical expectation, the oft-reported "warm glow" experienced by donors can be viewed as an opponent process in reaction to adverse emotional conditions (e.g., anxiety) before and during the initial donations. The B process appears to attenuate A state intensity with repeated donations, together with gradually increasing positive post-event affect.

Eating Behavior, Food Addiction, and a Modified Opponent Process Neurophysiology

If substances can be classified as potentially addictive based on the degree to which they evoke the release of dopamine, then food can certainly be added to cocaine, alcohol, nicotine, and many other substances as addictive. Indeed, it has been documented that dopamine levels in the body are elevated by the ingestion of chicken, turkey, fish, beef, soy, legumes, lettuce, spinach cabbage, cauliflower, broccoli, strawberries, green tea, olive oil, eggs, nuts, and coffee (among others) [10].

Researchers at Yale University have even constructed a 25-item food addiction scale based on criteria for addiction from the Diagnostic and Statistical Manual of Mental Disorders of the American Psychiatry Association [11]. It is a self-report inventory that includes items related to cravings for specific foods, eating more than planned, an increasing need for more food to feel satisfied, and importantly, physical, or psychological withdrawal symptoms such as irritability and anxiety when reducing food intake. What seems clear is that food has a dopaminergic effect that pertains to the same neurological reward pathways as substances of abuse [12].

Taken in the aggregate, it can be posited that the ingestion of foods with elevated dopaminergic properties may produce an affective disequilibrium with an elevated experience of pleasure, or the "A" state. The question remains as to whether the opponent process model of addictions fits the eating disorder literature, either in whole or in part. We can aver that at least in infrahuman research, the B process can be intense. Following food deprivation for example, rodents will display ravenous initial eating when food is made available. Further, rats subjected to a binge model of sucrose consumption show withdrawal-type symptoms when sucrose is removed; that is, tremors, teeth chattering, and head-shaking, as well as signs of rodent anxiety (e.g., complete cessation of motor activity; squeaking, hissing, increased heartrate). Perhaps analogous, albeit attenuated "B" conditions occur at the human level.

Opponent Process and Eating Behavior

Now, a brief review of opponent process principles that may be germane to this issue. First, if the food ingestion or "A" condition is dopaminergic and disruptive of homeostasis, then the opponent process “B” will be proportional but less intense. With succeeding ingestion, the dopaminergic effect will be less intense and closer to baseline as the “B” condition becomes stronger and its recruitment latency reduced. Craving, in the sense of overeating in an attempt to revivify the initial intensity of the A condition, is in accord with the Opponent Process mode. It is also important to note that the “B” condition will also be contiguously associated with neutral cues resulting in a type of Pavlovian conditioning. Such environmental conditioned stimuli can therefore evoke the “B” condition even in the absence of food ingestion.

Neurophysiology

Before continuing with food addiction and opponent process theory, we need to introduce some additional brain structures and functions to the neurophysiological model. The structures previously mentioned that constitute the reward circuitry include the nucleus accumbens (NAc) designated as the reward center. This is central to what Frank and colleagues at the University of California, San Diego [12] term the “dopamine receptor-mediated” network (Image 4.1) for hunger motivation and eating behavior. The network includes the nucleus accumbens as well as the ventral striatum (VS) and hypothalamus (see Image 4.1). The hypothalamus-VS circuity regulates the initiation and termination of eating behavior. It is also necessary to expand the demonstrable functions of the NAc in order to understand its role in possible food addiction. On the one hand, this reward center facilitates approach behaviors worthy of approbation; on the other hand, the NAc codes for avoidance behaviors, as a defense against outcomes that may be non-rewarding or aversive. It is also important to note that the NAc is located in and is part of the ventral striatum. This neurophysiological framework is central to our later chapter on practical implications (Chap. 8) that includes a section on the understanding and treatment of eating disorders.

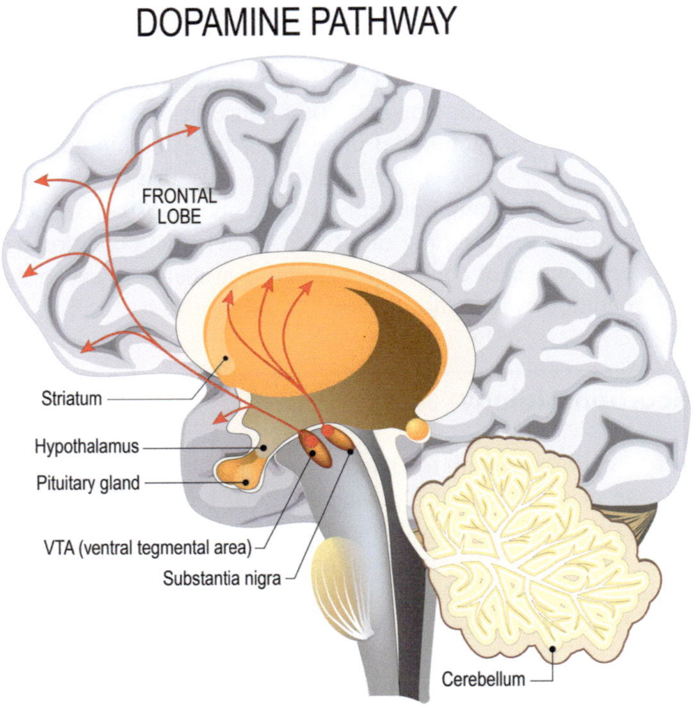

Image 4.1 Dopamine pathway. (Usage Rights Granted by IStock)

Test Anxiety

Perhaps most of the readership have experienced that vague fear state termed "anxiety" or "fear of failure," prior to completing an examination that will at least partially determine a classroom grade or an occupational decision. From an opponent process perspective, elevated negative affect of this type may be sufficiently intense to promote an hedonic contrast. Indeed, Craig and Siegel [13] administered a test of anxiety (the Mood Adjective Checklist) to 325 college students preceding a final course examination. A post-examination indicated demonstrated that congruent with Opponent Process Theory, negative affect does beget positive affect.

Breastfeeding

Data presented by Myers and Siegel [14] indicated that putting the baby to the breast is an exemplar of a positive emotional stimulus. This is juxtaposed to the removal of the infant from breast, producing a hedonic opposing condition. Women with current or previous breastfeeding experience completed retrospective emotionality ratings (Mood Adjective Checklist) reflecting various time periods before and during the breastfeeding process as well as during the weaning interval. The findings provided strong support of positive emotionality during nursing, mild dysphoria prior to a subsequent feeding schedule, and eventual reduced positive affect (habituation) consistent with opponent process theory.

Facial Afterimages

With a degree of hesitation, we conclude this chapter with reference to laboratory data on opponent afterimages of emotional facial expressions. We speculate there might be a real life, commonplace generalization of these data; it is interesting, but only a supposition. Research participants are required to visually fixate on the happy countenance of a pictured face. After a reasonable period of fixation, somewhat analogous to color afterimage research, the picture is removed and replaced by a face absent any emotional expressiveness. However, the prototypical participant will perceive and report contrasting emotional expressions such as sadness in response to the "neutral" visual stimulus. Or the converse if the fixation picture is one of anger or sadness. Here then, we are going beyond opponent processes pertaining to rods and cones and color perceptions to social phenomena [15]. It is hypothetically possible that interactions with a person or persons displaying very happy demeanors may engender an opposing emotional contrast effecting facial perceptions and perhaps social behaviors, but this is conjecture.

Autism Detour

An important consideration in this type of research is whether the participant veridically perceives the emotionality depicted in the initially observed facial configurations. The cognitive deficiency identified as "weak central coherence" in autism pertains to a perceptual focus on details without a corresponding capacity to integrate the details into a conceptual whole. Such a deficit might impede accurate recognition of facial patterns of emotionality. Indeed, when a single facial feature is exaggerated in a drawing, the person diagnosed with autism will tend to fixate on this detail to the detriment of an overall stimulus integration [16]. The weak central coherence likely occurs because of poor connectivity and synchronization among key brain centers [17]. And, indeed, afterimages inconsistent with OPT are found among individuals on the autism spectrum [18].

References

1. Ekkekakis P. The Dual-Mode Theory of affective responses to exercise in metatheoretical context: I. Initial impetus, basic postulates, and philosophical framework. Int Rev Sport Exerc Psychol. 2009;2(1):73–94. Available from: https://doi.org/10.1080/17509840802705920.
2. Schachter S, Singer J. Cognitive, social, and physiological determinants of emotional state. Psychol Rev. 1962;69(5):379–99. Available from: https://doi.org/10.1037/h0046234.
3. Markowitz SM, Arent SM. The exercise and affect relationship: evidence for the dual-mode model and a modified opponent process theory. J Sport Exerc Psychol. 2010;32(5):711–30. Available from: https://doi.org/10.1123/jsep.32.5.711.
4. Gaesser GA, Brooks G. A metabolic bases of excess post-exercise oxygen consumption. Med Sci Sports Exerc. 1984;16(1):29–43. Available from: https://doi.org/10.1249/00005768-198401000-00008.
5. Lochbaum M, Bixby W. Affect responses to acute bouts of aerobic exercise in fit and unfit participants: an examination of opponent-process theory. J Sport Behav. 2006;29:111–25.
6. Petruzzello S, Jones A, Tate A. Affective responses to acute exercise: a test of opponent-process theory. J Sports Med Phys Fitness. 1997;37(3):205–12. PMID: 9407752.

7. Landy FJ. An opponent process theory of job satisfaction. J Appl Psychol. 1978;63(5):533–47. Available from: https://doi.org/10.1037/0021-9010.63.5.533.
8. Bowling NA, Beehr TA, Wagner SH, Libkuman TM. Adaptation-level theory, opponent process theory, and dispositions: an integrated approach to the stability of job satisfaction. J Appl Psychol. 2005;90(6):1044–53. Available from: https://doi.org/10.1037/0021-9010.90.6.1044.
9. Piliavin JA, Callero PL, Evans DE. Addiction to altruism? Opponent-process theory and habitual blood donation. J Pers Soc Psychol. 1982;43(6):1200–13. Available from: https://doi.org/10.1037/0022-3514.43.6.1200.
10. Banyan Treatment Center. Dopamine foods boosting your mood naturally. n.d. Retrieved March 17, 2025, from Banyantreatmentcenter.com. https://www.banyantreatmentcenter.com/blog/dopamine-foods-boosting-your-mood-naturally/.
11. Gearhardt AN, Corbin WR, Brownell KD. Development of the Yale Food Addiction Scale version 2.0. Psychol Addict Behav. 2016;30(1):113–21. https://doi.org/10.1037/adb0000136. PMID: 26866783.
12. Frank GKW, Shott ME, DeGuzman MC. The neurobiology of eating disorders. Child Adolesc Psychiatr Clin N Am. 2019;28(4):629–40. Available from: https://doi.org/10.1016/j.chc.2019.05.007.
13. Craig RL, Siegel PS. Does negative affect beget positive affect? A test of the opponent-process theory. Bull Psychon Soc. 1979;14(6):404–6. Available from: https://doi.org/10.3758/bf03329492.
14. Myers HH, Siegel PS. The motivation to breastfeed: a fit to the opponent-process theory? J Pers Soc Psychol. 1985;49(1):188–93. Available from: https://doi.org/10.1037/0022-3514.49.1.188.
15. Russell JA, Fehr B. Relativity in the perception of emotion in facial expressions. J Exp Psychol Gen. 1987;116(3):223–37. Available from: https://doi.org/10.1037/0096-3445.116.3.223.
16. Rutherford MD, McIntosh DN. Rules versus prototype matching: strategies of perception of emotional facial expressions in the autism spectrum. J Autism Dev Disord. 2007;37(2):187–96. Available from: https://doi.org/10.1007/s10803-006-0151-9.
17. Peiker I, David N, Schneider TR, Nolte G, Schöttle D, Engel AK. Perceptual integration deficits in autism spectrum disorders are associated with reduced interhemispheric gamma-band coherence. J Neurosci. 2015;35(50):16352–61. Available from: https://doi.org/10.1523/jneurosci.1442-15.2015.
18. Rutherford MD, Troubridge EK, Walsh J. Visual afterimages of emotional faces in high functioning autism. J Autism Dev Disord. 2012;42(2):221–9. Available from: https://doi.org/10.1007/s10803-011-1233-x.

Criminology and Risk Motivation

5

Risk Motivation

"A life without risk is a life unlived," or some variation of the phrase, has historical antecedents derived from many philosophical, religious, and literary traditions, including the teachings of philosophers such as Aristotle [1] and Nietzsche [2]; Christian and Eastern theology [3, 4]; and ideas proposed by psychologists such as Jung and Maslow [5, 6]. The central principle of the phrase likely resonates with anyone possessing some foundational understanding of the nuances of life and human nature. After all, many of life's important experiences may never be without some degree of risk-taking. For example, a particularly risk-averse individual who might otherwise wish to find a romantic life partner may never do so if they are paralyzed by the potential hazards (e.g., rejection, embarrassment) that might come with asking someone out on a date. To that end, some level of risk must be beneficial for optimizing the human experience.

On the other hand, many risky behaviors are understandably maladaptive and hazardous in a more literal sense. For many of us, the act of committing a crime may represent the pinnacle of risky behavior. However, not all risky actions are necessarily criminal in nature. Be it drug abuse, self-inflicted injury, gam-

J. W. Gibson et al., *Opponent Process Theory*,
https://doi.org/10.1007/978-3-032-00090-3_5

bling, riding a bike without a helmet, or parachute jumping, there are a whole host of risky activities in which humans partake. We have all likely observed either in ourselves or others a willingness to engage in activities that present some affront to personal safety, emotional stability, financial security, and comforting certainty, although often with drastically varying degrees among different individuals. Why are some of us more likely than others to engage in risky activities? Attempts to explain such differences between individual proclivity to take risks—or to avoid them—have been the subject of research for quite some time. Various neurobiopsychosocial factors ranging from differing personality traits to variations in neurophysiology have been explored as potential underpinnings of risk-taking behavior.

Personality traits and their proposed biological and social bases have long been foundational to researching sensation-seeking and risk-taking behavior. The so-called "dimensions of personality" proposed by the German-born British psychologist Eysenck in the early-to-mid twentieth century served as the basis for numerous studies investigating links between differing personality types and tendencies for risk-taking behavior. These personality dimensions include "extraversion" (the degree to which an individual is social, active, and assertive), "neuroticism" (referring to emotional stability and a tendency to experience negative emotions such as depression and stress), and "psychoticism" (focusing on traits such as aggression, impulsiveness, and lack of empathy) [7]. Other personality traits proposed by Eysenck—"impulsiveness" and "venturesomeness" (the latter distinguished as a willingness to take risks for excitement or personal gain as opposed to sheer recklessness)—have been linked to higher measurements of psychoticism and extraversion, respectively [7, 8]. These findings informed the development of questionnaires such as the Eysenck Personality Inventory (EPI) and the Eysenck Personality Questionnaire (EPQ), which serve as measures of impulsiveness and venturesomeness.

Sensation Seeking Behavior

One of Eysenck's American counterparts, Zuckerman, would become known for his work exploring the biological and psychological framework of "sensation seeking," a trait he described as "the tendency to seek novel, varied, complex, and intense sensations and experiences and the willingness to take risks for the sake of such experiences" [9]. In 1964, Zuckerman and colleagues introduced the sensation seeking scale (SSS), a psychological tool for measuring individual differences in sensation seeking by exploring four separate subscales: thrill and adventure seeking, experience seeking, disinhibition, and boredom susceptibility [10]. The SSS has undergone multiple revisions, and its applications have been used to explore concepts such as the "optimal arousal hypothesis" (the proposal that sensation seekers have a higher optimal level of arousal than others) and the biological basis linking differences in neurotransmitter activity to differing degrees of impulsivity and the need for stimulation [11]. The SSS has been further used to study behavioral correlates such as extreme sports [12], reckless driving [13], gambling [14], drug use [15], alcohol consumption [16], risky sexual behavior [17, 18], preferences for exciting or intense forms of entertainment [19], creativity and openness to new experiences [20], and criminality and antisocial behavior [21].

Biological Correlations

While personality differences seem to play a role in different approaches to risk-taking behavior, the biology underlying motivation to engage in such behavior provides perhaps the most salient nexus between the aforementioned studies and potential application of opponent process theory. Studies have demonstrated that a variety of structural and physiological differences, including prefrontal cortex damage [22], reduced activity in the orbitofrontal cortex [23], higher levels of testosterone in men [24], lower levels of cortisol [25], and genetic heritability [26], are associated with increased sensation-seeking behaviors. Additionally, neurotransmitter function has been implicated. First, lower serotonin activity may be linked with poor decision-making and impulsivity [27]. On the other hand, dopamine has perhaps been investigated even more thoroughly. Increased dopamine transmission in certain brain regions, such as the ventral striatum [28], increased dopamine receptor density [29], and dopamine receptor gene polymorphisms [30], has been correlated with increased motivation to engage in novel, challenging, or stimulating activities.

Dopamine

Dopamine has often been implicated in the previously mentioned "optimal level of arousal hypothesis," given the central role of dopamine in the brain's reward system and its involvement in motivation, learning, and processing of novel stimuli [31–34]. The hypothesis itself posits that so-called "high sensation seekers" may have a lower baseline level of arousal or a higher threshold for stimulation, causing them to seek out more stimulating and novel experiences to achieve their optimal arousal level. This contrasts with so-called "low sensation seekers," who may have sufficient levels of dopamine activity such that they do not feel the need to seek out such intense experiences. These hypotheses have been empirically supported by studies assessing differences in individual SSS scores, physiological measures of arousal (e.g., heart rate, skin conductance, and cortisol levels) [35–39], and measurements of neurotransmitter activity [40–42] that correlate with varying preferences for and responses to high-stimulation and risky activity in both animal models and human subjects.

Homeostasis

In comparing the core underlying concepts of the optimal arousal hypothesis and the opponent process theory, we find a shared principle of balancing and regulating homeostasis. Early hypotheses that laid the groundwork for the idea of optimal arousal proposed that behavior is motivated by a need to maintain an optimal level of arousal and achieve a "psychological equilibrium" [43]. Considering the potential biological underpinnings we have discussed with regard to optimal arousal, we could reasonably postulate that the optimal arousal hypothesis represents an innate motivation to maintain homeostasis in response to endogenous alterations in physiology.

Opponent process theory, on the other hand, could instead be considered an acquired motivational drive to restore homeostasis in response to exogenous stimuli that essentially hijack our natural mechanisms for maintaining emotional and physiological balance. As first proposed by Solomon and Corbit [44], their expanded framework of the opponent process theorized that emotional states are regulated by two opposing processes. The first is the primary process (A-process), which is a direct response to a stimulus that may be pleasurable or aversive. The second is the opponent process (B-process), which is a compensatory response to counter the primary process in an effort to restore homeostasis. The final key component of the theory is that with repeated exposure to the initial stimulus, the A-process diminishes while the B-process strengthens over time. This theory has been applied to a variety of scenarios involving repetitive behaviors and the subsequent development of motivation to either lessen aversive responses or further engage in activities that promote pleasurable responses. These include risk-taking phenomena such as drug addiction [45, 46], skydiving and parachute jumping [44, 47], and nonsuicidal self-injury [48, 49].

Criminal Behavior

Although there has been far less investigation into any potential link between opponent process theory and criminal behavior, the theoretical exploration of at least some types of individuals who engage in criminal behavior through the lens of opponent process theory has been posited most notably by Rosellini and Lashley [50]. They presented an admittedly oversimplified and theoretical typological division between two groups of individuals who may engage in criminal behavior. One type of criminal was classified as "A-aversive" (referred to as "risk-averse" in this text for clarity): an individual with some extrinsic motivation to commit a crime who experiences anxiety, fear, and apprehension in response to the initial risk-taking stimulus of criminal activity but then experiences an opposing B-response of pleasant relief to counter the initial aversive reaction after completing the criminal act. The other type of criminal was classified as "A-pleasant" (referred to as "risk-embracing" in this text for clarity): an individual who experiences minimal fear and in fact may feel thrilled by the initial stimulus of a criminal act but then experience a counteracting aversive B-response after the crime (not unlike the craving someone might feel when they are withdrawing from a drug high).

In accordance with the final component of opponent process theory, these opposing types of criminals undergo different emotional changes with repeated exposure to criminal activity. Over time, the risk-averse criminal would experience less fear and anxiety with concurrent potentiation of the opposing sensation of relief such that it may strengthen even further to feelings of euphoria and excitement and thus perhaps embolden them to engage in further crime to sustain these newfound pleasurable after-effects. The risk-embracing criminal, on the other hand, would experience less of the initial thrill and instead endure worsening of the aversive counter response such that they may pursue even more criminal acts to achieve the initial "high" and stave off the "craving" sensation.

Opponent process theory also has potential implications for recidivism in the different types of criminals proposed by Rosellini and Lashley. In theory, if risk-averse criminals were to spend an extended period of time without committing any crimes, their homeostatic drive would reset to their baseline of fear and apprehension, thus making it less likely that they would engage in further criminal activity without a strong extrinsic motivating factor. However, if the same were to happen with the risk-embracing criminal, their homeostatic baseline would be reset to the initial thrill-seeking approach they have toward crime, and their propensity to engage in further criminal activity would be greater than that of the risk-averse individual. While Rosellini and Lashley acknowledge the heuristic nature of these theories, which do not necessarily account for many individuals who commit crime, they nonetheless raise intriguing questions about differing motivations between novice and experienced criminals regarding their initial and continued engagement in criminal behavior. Further empirical research on this subject may be fruitful in understanding at least one component of criminal motivation by measuring emotional and affective changes reported by individuals at different stages throughout their history of criminal activity.

In conclusion, it is exceedingly important to note that the topics discussed in this chapter do not consider a whole host of other factors that contribute to individuals' motivations to engage in risky behavior or criminal activity. The concepts of personality traits, biological differences, genetic variations, and theories of optimal arousal and the opponent process do not preclude the crucial impact on such behaviors by environmental factors, socioeconomic determinants, family dynamics, educational status, racial disparities, and cultural differences. Any holistic and useful understanding of the subject of risk-taking and criminal behavior should naturally account for all of these variables; the findings of extant and future research on the many different elements that play a role in these behaviors should be considered in combination as a whole to provide the most complete and constructive contribution to this area of study.

References

1. Aristotle. Nicomachean ethics. Translated by Ross WD. (c. 350 BCE). Available from: http://www.perseus.tufts.edu/hopper/.
2. Nietzsche F. Thus, spoke Zarathustra: a book for all and none. Translated by Kaufmann W. 1883. Penguin Classics; 1969.
3. The Bhagavad Gita. Translated by Easwaran E. (c. 500–200 BCE). Nilgiri Press; 2007.
4. The Dhammapada. Translated by Easwaran E. (c. 3rd century BCE). Nilgiri Press; 2007.
5. Jung C. The archetypes and the collective unconscious. Translated by Hull RFC. Princeton University Press; 1980.

6. Maslow A. Motivation and personality. Harper; 1954.
7. Eysenck HJ, Eysenck SBG. Personality and individual differences. Plenum Press; 1975.
8. Eysenck SBG, Eysenck HJ. Impulsiveness and venturesomeness: their position in a dimensional system of personality description. Psychol Rep. 1978;43(3_Suppl):1247–55. https://doi.org/10.2466/pr0.1978.43.3f.1247.
9. Zuckerman M. Behavioral expressions and biosocial bases of sensation seeking. Cambridge University Press; 1994.
10. Zuckerman M, Kolin EA, Price L, Zoob I. Development of a sensation-seeking scale. J Consult Psychol. 1964;28(6):477.
11. Zuckerman M. Sensation seeking: beyond the optimal level of arousal. Hillsdale: Lawrence Erlbaum Associates; 1979.
12. Zuckerman M. Sensation seeking and sports. Pers Individ Dif. 1983;4(3):285–93.
13. Jonah BA. Sensation seeking and risky driving: a review and synthesis of the literature. Accid Anal Prev. 1997;29(5):651–65.
14. Coventry KR, Brown RIF. Sensation seeking, gambling, and gambling addictions. Addiction. 1993;88(4):541–54.
15. Zuckerman M, Ball S, Black J. Influences of sensation seeking, gender, risk appraisal, and situational factors on smoking behavior. J Pers Soc Psychol. 1990;57(5):992–1002.
16. Hittner JB, Swickert R. Sensation seeking and alcohol use: a meta-analytic review. Addict Behav. 2006;31(8):1383–401.
17. Zuckerman M, Eysenck SBG, Eysenck HJ. Sensation seeking in England and America: cross-cultural, age, and sex comparisons. J Consult Clin Psychol. 1978;46(1):139–49.
18. Hoyle RH, Fejfar MC, Miller JD. Personality and sexual risk taking: a quantitative review. J Pers. 2000;68(6):1203–31.
19. Zuckerman M. Sensation seeking and reactions to media violence. J Commun. 1988;38(3):29–45.
20. Martindale C, Dailey A. Creativity, primary process cognition, and personality. Pers Individ Dif. 1996;20(4):409–14.
21. Horvath P, Zuckerman M. Sensation seeking, risk appraisal, and risky behavior. Pers Individ Dif. 1993;14(1):41–52.
22. Bechara A, Damasio H, Damasio AR, Anderson SW. Deciding advantageously before knowing the advantageous strategy. Science. 2001;275(5306):1293–5.
23. Knoch D, Gianotti LR, Baumgartner T, Fehr E. The role of the orbitofrontal cortex in social behavior. Trends Cogn Sci. 2006;14(1):10–5.
24. Dabbs JM, Morris R. Testosterone and occupational choice: the importance of risk-taking. Pers Individ Dif. 1990;12(3):248–56.
25. Fowles DC. The three psychophysiological substrates of personality. Psychophysiology. 1980;17(2):51–64.

26. Zuckerman M, Kuhlman DM. Personality and risk-taking: common biosocial factors. J Pers. 2000;68(6):999–1029.
27. Kuepper Y, Grant P, Wielpuetz C, Hennig J. The role of serotonin in the neurobiological basis of personality traits. J Neurosci. 2010;30(31):10592–600.
28. Zuckerman M, Joireman J, Kraft M, Kuhlman DM. Sensation seeking and dopaminergic function. Biol Psychol. 1993;37(2):123–35.
29. Depue RA, Collins PF. Neurobiology of the structure of personality: dopamine, facilitation of incentive motivation, and extraversion. Behav Brain Sci. 1999;22(4):491–517.
30. Ebstein RP, Novick O, Umansky R, Priel B, Osher Y, Blaine D, et al. Dopamine D4 receptor (DRD4) gene polymorphism and novelty seeking in humans. Nat Genet. 1996;12(1):78–80.
31. Wise RA. Dopamine, learning, and motivation. Nat Rev Neurosci. 2004;5(6):483–94. https://doi.org/10.1038/nrn1406.
32. Schultz W, Dayan P, Montague PR. A neural substrate of prediction and reward. Science. 1997;275(5306):1593–9. https://doi.org/10.1126/science.275.5306.1593.
33. Berridge KC, Robinson TE. Dopamine and reward: parsing the data. Trends Neurosci. 1998;21(9):371–7. https://doi.org/10.1016/S0166-2236(98)01340-9.
34. Kakade S, Dayan P. Dopamine: generalization and novelty. Neural Comput. 2002;14(5):1095–113. https://doi.org/10.1162/089976602753712918.
35. Zuckerman M. Sensation seeking and the endogenous deficit theory of drug abuse. NIDA Res Monogr. 1986;74:59–70. Available from: https://books.google.com/books?hl=en&id=hGyonlYcaFEC.
36. Wilson LC, Scarpa A. Aggressive behavior and resting heart rate: a meta-analytic review. Aggress Behav. 2011;37(4):269–80. Available from: https://onlinelibrary.wiley.com/doi/abs/10.1002/ab.20369.
37. Coventry KR, Constable B. Physiological arousal and sensation-seeking in female fruit machine gamblers. Addiction. 1999;94(3):425–30. Available from: https://onlinelibrary.wiley.com/doi/abs/10.1046/j.1360-0443.1999.94342512.x.
38. Zuckerman M. Biosocial bases of sensation seeking. In: Biology of personality and individual differences. The Guilford Press; 2006. Available from: https://www.academia.edu/download/99399686/Biology_of_Personality_and_Individual_Differences_Turhan_Canli_.pdf#page=56.
39. Herman AM, Critchley HD, Duka T. The role of emotions and physiological arousal in modulating impulsive behaviour. Biol Psychol. 2018;133:30–43. Available from: https://www.sciencedirect.com/science/article/pii/S0301051118300644.
40. Blanchard RD, Blanchard DC. The neural basis of animal aggression. J Int Neuropsychol Soc. 2003;9(5):899–907.

41. Manuck SB, Flory JD, Muldoon MF, Ferrell RE. Neurotransmitter function and aggression. Biol Psychiatry. 2003;53(2):131–40.
42. Zald DH, Cowan RL, Riccardi P, Baldwin RM, Ansari MS, Li R, et al. Dopamine transmission in the striatum is associated with sensation seeking. Nat Neurosci. 2008;11(6):725–7.
43. Hebb DO. Drives and the C.N.S. (conceptual nervous system). Psychol Rev. 1955;62(4):243–54.
44. Solomon RL, Corbit JD. An opponent-process theory of motivation: I. Temporal dynamics of affect. Psychol Rev. 1974;81(2):119–45. Available from: https://psycnet.apa.org/record/1974-26855-001.
45. Solomon RL. Addiction: an opponent-process theory of acquired motivation: the affective dynamics of addiction. Psychol Rev. 1977;84(2):119–45. Available from: https://psycnet.apa.org/record/1992-98221-002.
46. Berridge KC, Robinson TE. Addiction and incentive-sensitization. Psychopharmacology. 2016;236(9):2721–56. Available from: https://doi.org/10.1007/s00213-016-4215-5.
47. Epstein S. Toward a unified theory of anxiety. Prog Exp Pers Res. 1967;4:133–72. Available from: https://pubmed.ncbi.nlm.nih.gov/4867096/.
48. Solomon RL. The opponent-process theory of acquired motivation: the costs of pleasure and the benefits of pain. Am Psychol. 1980;35(8):691–712.
49. Franklin JC, Hessel ET, Aaron RV, Arthur MS, Heilbron N, Prinstein MJ. The functions of nonsuicidal self-injury: support for cognitive-affective regulation and opponent processes from a novel psychophysiological paradigm. J Abnorm Psychol. 2010;119(4):850–62.
50. Rosellini RA, Lashley RL. Opponent-process theory: implications for criminality. In: McCord J, editor. Facts, frameworks, and forecasts. 1st ed. New York: Routledge; 1992. p. 55–76.

Pain Relief, Self-inflicted Injuries, and Acupuncture

6

Pain

Pain is physical discomfort on a continuum of mild to severe. Pain is related to some form of tissue damage detected by nerves called nociceptors. A overly simplified neurophysiology of pain is (a) detection followed by (b) transmission and (c) arrival at the cerebral pain center, the insular cortex.

Pain Relief

Research on pain reduction often begins with a thermal pain stimulus. With rodents, for example, radiant heat from a focused beam of light is applied to the hind paws. Human participants a heat stimulus may be applied to the back of the hand.

Leknes et al. [1] investigated the following hypotheses pertaining to the infliction of pain and the consequences following termination of the painful stimulus:

1. Relief from pain is an opponent process.
2. Relief from an unpleasant sensation such as pain is always less intense than the unpleasant sensation itself; and it is weaker and slower than the original unpleasant stimulus.
3. Therefore, as stated above, relief is always less intense than the stimulus that is unpleasant, such as pain.

J. W. Gibson et al., *Opponent Process Theory*,
https://doi.org/10.1007/978-3-032-00090-3_6

4. The degree of relief is related to the speed of termination of the unpleasant stimulus such as pain.
5. The opponent process to pain is rewarding.

In a series of experiments with humans, the investigation found that (a) the mean pain level ratings were significantly higher than the mean relief measure; (b) both the intensity of pain and the intensity of relief increased sequentially; (c) relief from pain is rewarding; and (d), one's sense of relief is correlated with the attenuation or cessation of the painful stimulus, but pain reduction and relief are not synonymous.

It is important to note that this study dealt entirely with acute pain. A generalization of findings to long-term or chronic pain manifestations cannot be made. Nevertheless, the Leknes et al.'s [1] research was well-conducted (internally valid) and included three separate investigations, and to date, it is an exemplary study testing hypotheses generated from opponent process theory. A point of emphasis in this study is item "d" above, the non-equivalence of pain-stimulus removal and the experience of relief: Ratings of pain relief are not equal to a diminution of pain stimulus intensity. From an opponent process perspective, relief occurs with the advent of the hedonic contrast, from pain related anxiety to the pleasantry of relief. Similar findings were later reported with a cold presser pain stimulus [2]. Pain and pleasurable relief are reciprocal, interacting opponents.

In two investigations, [2, 3] discuss the neurological underpinning of pain and opponent pleasure in relation to brain structures and endogenous brain chemicals. While acknowledging the role of the ventral striatum and dopamine in pleasurable relief, these investigators further implicate the orbitofrontal cortex and endogenous opioids in the opponent reaction to pain stimuli. Moreover, the authors provide functional neuroimaging data in support of opponent interactions. Specifically, a noxious stimulus activates several neuro-structures including the thalamus and insula, while simultaneously de-activating areas of the orbitofrontal cortex and the release of endogenous opioids as well as altering ventral striatal functioning and dopamine release. Noxious stimulus interruption or withdrawal results in a re-activation.

It should be mentioned that there are two types of endogenous opioids related to pain and opponent processes (we will classify them with "abstruse complexity" as bad and good). Dynorphins are "bad" in the sense of being correlated with negative emotional conditions and pain. Endorphins are the "good" opioids associated with pain reduction and mood elevation. It is noteworthy that dynorphin release is an initial biochemical reaction to painful thermal stimuli and may also relate to the biochemistry of acupuncture [4].

Note on Pain Placebos

To our knowledge, studies on possible opponent aftereffects of analgesic placebos have not been implemented, though the mechanisms that underpin placebo effectiveness seem to follow the same neurophysiological circuitry as depicted in the OPT emotionally elevating A condition. The possible hedonic contrast to placebo induction might be a fruitful area of research.

An investigation by Ellingsen et al. [5] is illuminating in this regard. Participants were administered an inert nasal spray with the expectation that "oxytocin" in the nasal spray could reduce the unpleasantness of an impending painful touch. Functional magnetic resonance imaging (FMRI) data indicated that the effectiveness of the "oxytocin" in pain attenuation was related to activation of the dopaminergic reward system involving the NAc and VTA. Alternatively, perhaps the dopaminergic effect was related to an independent opponent hedonic contrast; or conceivably, placebo expectations and OPT reactions might have an interacting combined impact.

Self-inflicted Injuries (Non-suicidal Self-injury or NSSI; Also Termed Self-inflicted Behavior, or SIB)

Perhaps, it is fair to say that for most humans, there is a desire for pleasure to be maximized and pain minimized. Why then are there subgroups who voluntarily appear to violate this aphorism? An attractive feature of opponent process theory is its potential for rendering a seemingly incomprehensible behavioral actions such as self-inflicted pain, intelligible. The simple hypothesized motivation to engage in repeated self-injuries is the positive hedonic aftereffect. Nevertheless, opponent process theory is but one of several explanatory constructs for non-suicidal self-injuries that require further investigation.

There is no question that NSSI constitute a major problem in our society especially with adolescents. A recent world-wide meta-analysis included 62 independent investigations and 264,638 adolescent participants, across a 2010–2021 time period. The findings indicated that 20.3% of the adolescents were involved in repetitive NSSI, while another 8.3% engaged in episodic self-injuries [6].

NSSI and Opponent Process Theory

In a 2015 literature review [7], the investigators reported that both the control participants and persons with a history of non-suicidal self-injurious behaviors responded to experiment-applied noxious stimuli in a similar mood regulation fashion. Consistent with the pain study of Leknes [1], the induction of pain and its termination are followed by pleasurable relief. Further, in studies asking NSSI participants to visualize and imagine engaging in an NSSI act, there was a subsequent declivity of negative affect. However, no evidence was found for a gradual increase in the strength of a positive opponent process, albeit there was a dearth of studies in the review designed to evaluate the hedonic contrast across multiple time periods.

Endogenous Opioids

The discovery of the endogenous opioid system was a remarkable step toward understanding analgesic mechanisms and may be germane in fostering research on the perplexing antecedents of NSSI.

Again, with focus on the opponent process, one ascending hypothesis in the etiology of self-injuries involves the release of endogenous opioids in response to pain, more specifically the Beta-endorphin and enkephalins. The opioid peptide B-endorphin reportedly reduces pain, whereas enkephalins are implicated in the regulation of pain sensations; in addition, both opioids pertain to affect regulation. The literature review by Bresin and Gordon [8] corroborates the posited release of these opioid peptides in response to pain. This is based on findings of increased levels of these endogenous opioids following self-injuries together with data indicating positive effects of opioid antagonists as treatment modalities.

Acupuncture

There are also conflicting data on the equivalence of manual versus electrical modes of stimulation. What we do know is that acupuncture is an approach of traditional Chinese medicine that originated over two millennia ago. And according to a recent literature review [9], since 1975, there have been over 10,000 randomized controlled studies on acupuncture, together with 2471 systematic reviews on the topic from world-wide researchers, mainly from China, the United States, and the United Kingdom. The authors proclaimed that indeed acupuncture has demonstrated effectiveness across numerous dysfunctions including the reduction of pain. On the other hand, Paley and Johnson [10] concluded that the systematic reviews of acupuncture data on pain attenuation have methodological flaws and are at best, inconclusive. The acronym AMSTAR refers to "A Measurement Tool to Assess Systematic Reviews"; it provides criteria for evaluating the adequacy of literature reviews. Based on the standards of AMSTAR 2, Ji et al. [11] concluded that the methodological quality of reviews on acupuncture is deficient, especially in failure to include studies with negative findings.

So, despite prodigious, decades long research productivity that includes cross-cultural investigations and randomized controlled studies, the efficacy of acupuncture as a treatment modality may still be in dispute.

Hypothesized Analgesic Biochemistry

Dynorphins are evoked by acupuncture, at least with high frequency electroacupuncture stimulation [12]. Assuming acupuncture effectiveness, dynorphins activate the OPT anti-reward system since they reduce dopaminergic output in the nucleus accumbens. Acupuncture can also increase GABA-mediated synaptic transmission that may in turn combine with dynorphins to further reduce dopaminergic functions. In the aggregate, it is hypothesized that certain elevated frequency levels of electroacupuncture promote an adverse A condition, mainly related to the combined effects of dynorphins and GABA and set into motion the compensatory B state.

Conflicting Data on Dynorphins

Indeed, there is evidence that dynorphins are the "bad" endogenous opioids, associated with hyperalgesia, stress, and adverse emotional conditions [13–16]. Conversely there are also contradictory data, indicating dynorphins may evince a salubrious, analgesic impact [12, 17]. Thus, there is a controversy: Are dynorphins involved in promoting or relieving pain?

Conflict Resolution? The OPT Hypothesis

Perhaps from an opponent process perspective, there is no controversy-dynorphins promote hyperanalgesia and negative emotional states (condition A) that antedates emergence of an analgesic, relief state (condition B). More specifically, dynorphins (and GABA) may activate the anti-reward system, beginning with a reduction of dopamine output in the nucleus accumbens. This anti-reward hyperanalgesic system is then countered with activation of the reward system that in pain relief includes the release of "good" endogenous opioids. Perhaps future research will attempt to refute this hypothesis.

In sum, the information in this chapter suggests a reasonable, but certainly not absolute "fit" between induced pain and compensatory opponent effects. Pain relief and hedonic contrasts require biochemical modifications to the basic OPT formulations together with relevant additional research.

References

1. Leknes S, Brooks JCW, Wiech K, Tracey I. Pain relief as an opponent process: a psychophysical investigation. Eur J Neurosci. 2008;28(4):794–801. Available from: https://doi.org/10.1111/j.1460-9568.2008.06380.x.
2. Bitar N, Marchand S, Potvin S. Pleasant pain relief and inhibitory conditioned pain modulation: a psychophysical study. Pain Res Manag. 2018;2018:1–8. Available from: https://doi.org/10.1155/2018/1935056.
3. Bitar N, Dugré JR, Marchand S, Potvin S. Medial orbitofrontal deactivation during tonic cold pain stimulation: a fMRI study examining the opponent-process theory. J Pain Res. 2020;13:1335–47. Available from: https://doi.org/10.2147/jpr.s248056.
4. Massaly N. Pain-induced negative affect is mediated via recruitment of the nucleus accumben kappa opioid system. J Pain. 2019;20(4):S62. Available from: https://doi.org/10.1016/j.jpain.2019.02.045.
5. Ellingsen D-M, Wessberg J, Eikemo M, Liljencrantz J, Endestad T, Olausson H, et al. Placebo improves pleasure and pain through opposite modulation of sensory processing. Proc Natl Acad Sci USA. 2013;110(44):17993–8. Available from: https://doi.org/10.1073/pnas.1305050110.
6. Xiao Q, Song X, Huang L, Hou D, Huang X. Global prevalence and characteristics of non-suicidal self-injury between 2010 and 2021 among a non-clinical sample of adolescents: a meta-analysis. Front Psychiatry. 2022;13:912441. Available from: https://doi.org/10.3389/fpsyt.2022.912441.
7. Hamza CA, Willoughby T. Nonsuicidal self-injury and affect regulation: recent findings from experimental and ecological momentary assessment studies and future directions. J Clin Psychol. 2015;71(6):561–74. Available from: https://doi.org/10.1002/jclp.22174.

8. Bresin K, Gordon KH. Endogenous opioids and nonsuicidal self-injury: a mechanism of affect regulation. Neurosci Biobehav Rev. 2013;37(3):374–83. Available from: https://doi.org/10.1016/j.neubiorev.2013.01.020.
9. Lu L, Zhang Y, Tang X, Ge S, Wen H, Zeng J, et al. Evidence on acupuncture therapies is underused in clinical practice and health policy. BMJ. 2022;376:e067475. Available from: https://doi.org/10.1136/bmj-2021-067475.
10. Paley CA, Johnson MI. Acupuncture for the relief of chronic pain: a synthesis of systematic reviews. Medicina. 2019;56(1):6. Available from: https://doi.org/10.3390/medicina56010006.
11. Ji Z, Zhang J, Menniti-Ippolito F, Massari M, Fauci AJ, Li N, et al. The quality of Cochrane systematic reviews of acupuncture: an overview. BMC Complement Med Ther. 2020;20(1):307. Available from: https://doi.org/10.1186/s12906-020-03099-9.
12. Han J-S. Acupuncture and endorphins. Neurosci Lett. 2004;361(1–3):258–61. Available from: https://doi.org/10.1016/j.neulet.2003.12.019.
13. Caudle RM, Mannes AJ. Dynorphin: friend or foe? Pain. 2000;87(3):235–9. Available from: https://doi.org/10.1016/s0304-3959(00)00360-2.
14. Laughlin TM, Larson AA, Wilcox GL. Mechanisms of induction of persistent nociception by dynorphin. J Pharmacol Exp Ther. 2001;299(1):6–11. Available from: https://doi.org/10.1016/s0022-3565(24)29295-8.
15. Ito H, Navratilova E, Vagnerova B, Watanabe M, Kopruszinski C, Moreira de Souza LH, et al. Chronic pain recruits hypothalamic dynorphin/kappa opioid receptor signaling to promote wakefulness and vigilance. Brain. 2023;146(3):1186–99. Available from: https://doi.org/10.1093/brain/awac153.
16. Hang A, Wang Y, He L, Liu J. The role of the dynorphin/κ opioid receptor system in anxiety. Acta Pharmacol Sin. 2015;36(7):783–90. Available from: https://doi.org/10.1038/aps.2015.32.
17. Costigan M, Woolf CJ. No dream, no pain. Cell. 2002;108(3):297–300. Available from: https://doi.org/10.1016/s0092-8674(02)00640-2.

Learning, Motivation, and Opponent Process Theory

7

Ivan Pavlov: Pavlovian or Classical Conditioning

Learning can be defined as a process by which an activity originates or is changed, provided that the origin or change cannot be accounted for by temporary conditions (e.g., drug conditions) or maturation [1].

There is a type of learning that humans share with virtually all-living creatures, including the amoeba, insects, and even bacteria. It begins with the presentation of a stimulus, defined as anything that produces activity in a sensory organ. As you will probably recall, Ivan Pavlov, the pioneering Russian physiologist, presented food powder to a hungry dog. The food powder naturally evoked salivation. Next, he paired (i.e., associated contiguously in time, usually within 5 s) a stimulus with the food powder that had no "power" in relation to producing salivation, the sound of a bell. This was the sequence:

$$\text{Bell} \rightarrow \text{Food powder} \rightarrow \text{Salivation}$$

After many repetitions of this sequence, the food powder was removed. Now presentation of the Bell alone was followed by the salivation response.

J. W. Gibson et al., *Opponent Process Theory*,
https://doi.org/10.1007/978-3-032-00090-3_7

Bell → Salivation

This indeed constitutes a change in behavior, consistent with our definition of learning; the dog acquired a response to a new stimulus. In Pavlovian terms, the food powder was initially an unconditioned or unlearned stimulus (UCS) that elicited an unlearned, innate response. The bell was initially a neutral stimulus (neutral or powerless to effect salivation); through learning via repeated association in time, the bell became a learned or conditioned stimulus (CS); salivation in response to the bell alone became the learned or conditioned response (CR) [2, 3].

Image 7.1 is an illustration that begins with the sight and aroma of food as the unconditioned or unlearned stimulus defined as the stimulus that naturally or innately produces salivation.

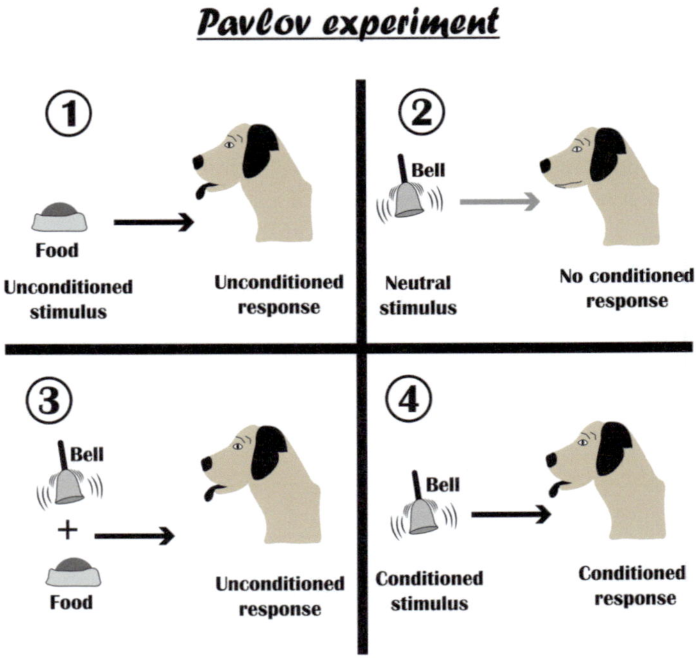

Image 7.1 Classical conditioning. (Usage Rights Granted by IStock)

In humans, Pavlovian conditioning involves the autonomic or involuntary nervous system. The responses mediated by the autonomic nervous system (ANS) are typically not under voluntary control. The ANS is the system that controls pupil dilation and constriction, heart rate, salivation, and importantly and is involved in emotional reactions. The unlearned stimulus can be either positive or aversive. *The cardinal point is that when we learn a new stimulus-response connection (and the response is mediated by the ANS), the body responds automatically when the learned stimulus is present. It is involuntary.* These so-called classically conditioned behaviors are called respondents [4].

Pavlov

Pavlov also experimented with dogs in a manner congruent with subsequent expositions of opponent process theory. For instance, he placed the animal in a harness that prevented escape and then exposed the dog to an electric shock as the unconditioned stimulus. The aversive stimulus produced an A state characterized by heart rate acceleration as well as behaviors interpreted as terror and panic. When the shock terminated after 10 s, the animal appeared subdued and inhibited and the cardiac rate decelerated. With repeated shock trials, the B emotional state was described as joyful over time; importantly, a neutral stimulus associated with shock could elicit the B emotional and behavioral consequences later, via Pavlovian conditioning [5].

Other Examples

1. On the human level, a medication that kills cancer cells also causes nausea. When a cancer patient associates the injection syringe for the medication with impending nausea, over time just the sight of the syringe produces involuntary nausea.
2. The presentation of a large, bright yellow lemon causes your lips to automatically pucker.

3. You enter an empty auditorium where earlier you experienced performance anxiety when attempting to deliver a speech to the large, assembled crowd. Even though no human beings are present, the empty chairs, the podium, and other formerly neutral stimuli evoke panic because of Pavlovian conditioning (and perhaps a subsequent B condition).

More germane to our discussion is the documented fact that when we experience extreme emotional arousal, cues (neutral stimuli) present in the environment become associated with that arousal and can become conditioned stimuli for that emotional state and perhaps the opposing hedonic contrast (more about this below). Importantly, cognitions (mental images; covert self-speech) can become conditioned stimuli that elicit ANS-mediated responses.

For example, imagine sitting at your kitchen table staring at a large, brightly colored lemon. You then cut the lemon in half and then in quarters. You take one of the four juicy lemon slices into your mouth and bite into the exceedingly sour fibrous core. For most of us, this imaginary encounter will result in an actual salivation experience.

In the above Pavlovian example, the imagined taste of a sour lemon resulted in the unconditioned or unlearned experience, with the sour taste (UCS) eliciting salivation (UCR). At the same time, the words "lemon" and "sour" were likely used as verbal labels associated with the taste-sour-salivation experience and thus became conditioned stimuli (CS) in relation to the ANS mediated salivation. Now, reading or hearing phrases that include "sour" and "lemon" as in the story above can possibly evoke the CR of salivation, all with imaginary visual and taste imagery.

It is also important to mention that the human cognitive abilities for classification and concept formation can expand the generalization of Pavlovian learning. If, for instance, words such as apple, peach, and pear are independently conditioned to the blinking response to a puff of air to the eyeball, hearing or reading the words separately will elicit blinking behavior, but so too will a classification term "fruit," a word that was never directly a part of Pavlovian learning [6–9].

Unlearning of Pavlovian Responses or Extinction

Behaviors learned through the process of Pavlovian conditioning can be helpful and adaptive or harmful and maladaptive to the individual. Pavlov also investigated the unlearning of responses or what has come to be known as *extinction*. Recall that the bell (NS) must be contiguously associated within a brief time period with the food powder (US) in order for simple classical conditioning to occur. It can be stated that at least in principle, the food powder is desirable and rewarding to the organism, and that salivation is indeed strengthened by the presence of the food powder. When the food powder is removed following repeated trials, so too is the strengthen mechanism. The Bell → Salivation connection will not continue indefinitely. Following repeated presentations of the bell absent food powder, the CR (salivation) will eventually fail to occur. This is termed extinction. The reintroduction of the US will revivify the CR. However, as will be discussed later, extinction of undesirable CRs can be the goal of certain therapeutic interventions [4].

Aversive Pavlovian Conditioning

A hospitalized patient diagnosed with "alcoholism" is administered emetine, a chemical that induces nausea. As the patient begins to experience the aversive effects of emetine, she/he is taken to a treatment room in which the patient's favorite alcoholic beverage is poured into a large glass. The patient begins with olfactory stimulation, smelling the beverage. As the nausea continues to increase in intensity, the patient then tastes to beverage and then ingests copious amounts. This is followed by regurgitation into a container and engages again in olfactory stimulation (smelling the emesis). This is repeated several times each alternate day session for 2 weeks. The typical result is that the smell and taste of the beverage evokes nausea, in the absence of the emetine. Importantly, neutral cues associated with "aversion therapy" also elicited nausea [10].

Skinnerian or Operant Learning

Ivan Pavlov and Burrhus Frederic (B. F.) Skinner are the two major figures in the field of learning. Unlike Pavlov, Skinner dealt with responses mediated by the "voluntary," not the autonomic nervous system. Thus, his interests were not in automatic physiological responses but in the learning of controllable, voluntary behaviors. He used the term "operant" to refer to such behaviors, meaning that the organism actually learns to "operate" voluntarily on objects in the environment in order to produce desired outcomes or avoid and escape negative ones [11].

In operant conditioning, unlike Pavlovian learning, the operant response comes *before* the stimulus, to wit:

$$\begin{aligned} &\mathit{Response}\left(\text{e.g., voluntarily telling a joke}\right) \\ &\rightarrow \mathit{Stimulus}\left(\text{e.g., group laughter}\right) \end{aligned}$$

George tells a joke for the first time, and it engenders laughter. The next time George is in a social setting, he tells several jokes, each of which evokes laughter. The laughter can be defined as a *reinforcer*, meaning, in this instance, a social stimulus (laughter), a secondary reinforcer that strengthens (increases the frequency of) the preceding action.

In Skinner's approach to learning the association is between the action and its consequences. In Image 7.2, a *positive* reinforcer (as in our example) is typically something pleasant that follows the action. A *negative* reinforcer is something aversive that is removed after an action resulting, like any reinforcer, in a strengthening of the response. Negative reinforcement is not punishment, although the two are often confused. A *punisher* is an aversive consequence of an action that weakens the response (Image 7.3). Importantly, a given aversive stimulus can be a negative reinforcer (when removed) or a punisher (when presented) [11].

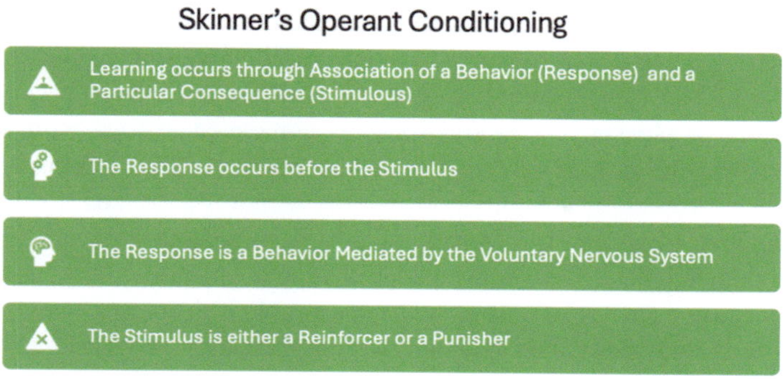

Image 7.2 Stimulus, response, and learning. (Usage Rights Granted by IStock)

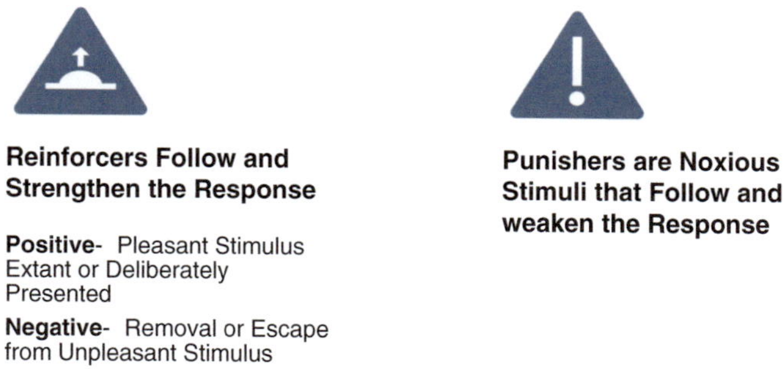

Image 7.3 Reinforcers and punishers. (Usage Rights Granted by IStock

Interactions Between Classical and Operant Learning [12–14]

It may not be intuitively obvious, but food itself can be both an unconditioned stimulus for Pavlov (i.e., it naturally elicits autonomic nervous system responses such as salivation) and a positive reinforcer for Skinner (i.e., it can strengthen a voluntary behavior). For example, if food is presented before a response, the sight and smell will elicit pupil dilation and salivation automatically. If food is presented after a voluntary nervous system response, it will potentially strengthen or reinforce the preceding behavioral act. A *primary reinforcer* to Skinner is something that satisfies a "need" or "want" state; that is, it is something necessary for survival or pleasure. A neutral stimulus associated in time with a primary reinforcer may, in a Pavlovian sense, acquire reinforcement properties; when this occurs, the stimulus is termed a *secondary reinforcer*. Money has no inherent rewarding characteristics; it is simply paper or a small metallic alloy. But because of its relationship with pleasurable objects that satisfy needs and wants, it acquires powerful secondary reinforcement properties. Voluntary nervous system behaviors maintained by positive or negative reinforcement are termed operants.

Primary and Secondary Reinforcers

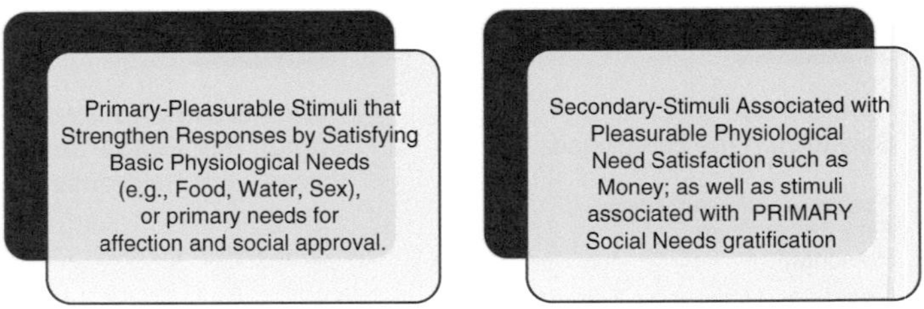

There are two *operants* germane to understanding of opponent process theory. Both relate to unpleasant (aversive) stimuli. In *escape* learning, the aversive stimulus is present, and the operant behavior is effective in removing or allowing the person to be physically removed from the stimulus. In *avoidance* learning, the operant behavior allows the person not to encounter the aversive stimulus at all. The sequence of behaviors that is successful in avoiding something that might be unpleasant or painful become reinforcing. This means that by not directly facing an aversive event via avoidance or escape, the behaviors become energized and strengthened and will likely be repeated in the future with similar contingencies [15–17].

Example of Avoidance Learning

A rodent is placed in a Skinner box, similar to the one in Image 7.4, and subjected to an electric shock in an electrified grid. However, a light (visual stimulus) is presented 10 s before the onset of the noxious stimulus. The 10 s time period will allow the rodent to engage in a voluntary behavior, moving outside the electrical grid, to avoid the noxious stimulus. How many trials will take place before the rodent responds to the light and learns to avoid the noxious stimulus. And if the animal eventually avoids

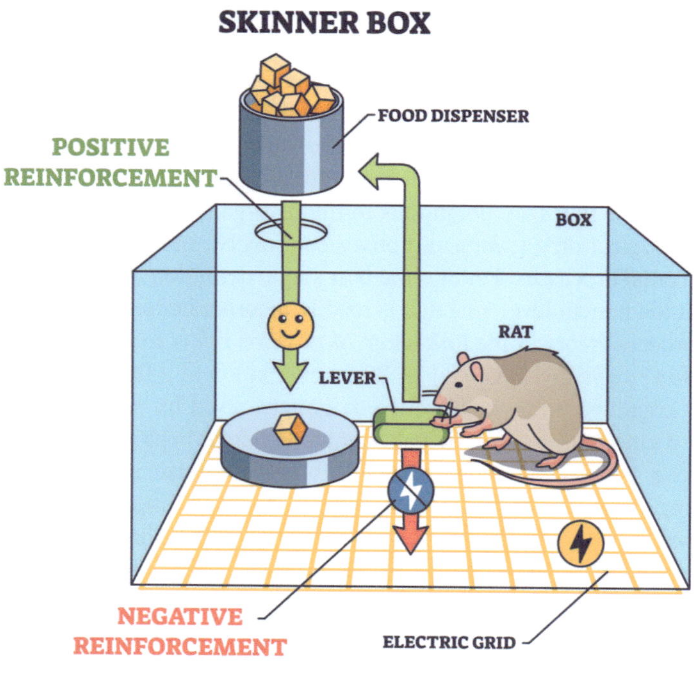

Image 7.4 Skinner box. (Usage Rights Granted by IStock)

the shock by escaping from the grid, upon return to the Skinner box and the same procedures, will the rat immediately respond to the visual stimulus that signals impending pain and circumvent the electric shock entirely. This is avoidance learning.

Motivation and OPT

Opponent process theory (OPT) also subsumes the construct of "motivation." In fact, it is often described as a theory of acquired motivation. The etymology of the word "motivation" begins with the Latin "movere," meaning "to move." A motive is a spring to action; it involves the activation of behavior. At the most basic level, motives are the "drives" that "push" the individual into action [18]. These are the irritating biological deficits or needs, such as hunger and thirst that actuate and direct behavior toward goals that will reduce the drive state by satisfying need for something necessary for survival and enhancing the stimulus value of events associated with need satisfaction (e.g., supermarkets; drinking fountains). Although not necessary for survival, an irritating B condition in OPT can be viewed as an acquired drive or "push" motive that is necessary for adaptation.

Drive states are ubiquitous for living organisms. In addition to biological drives, human motives can involve more complicated mental processes. Perhaps the best single definition of motivation at the human level, one that is readily incorporated into opponent process theory, is the following: *Motivation refers to the* ***anticipation*** *of affective change* [19, 20]. Anticipation of a future event is a cognitive process. Affective is the term used by psychologists for emotion. If one anticipates that a particular behavior will lead to a positive emotional change, this will arouse and energize engagement in that behavior. If the individual anticipates that a behavior will lead to a negative emotional change, there is arousal related to avoiding this behavioral act. These are the future anticipated conditions that "pull" the individual into activity. In OPT, for example, when the A state is aversive, the hedonic after effect may become an anticipated acquired motive.

Specifics of OPT Motivation

The A condition can be pleasurable or aversive; both emotional states have somewhat different motivational dynamics. When pleasurable to the point of producing disequilibrium, it is an emotional negative after effect that "pushes" or drives the individual into action and contingent operants. The positive A condition adheres to our definition of motivation, "the anticipation of a positive change in affect" that impels and energizes action. The B state, or hedonic contrast, constitutes an irritant that pushes or drives the individual in directions that will provide reduction or escape from the aversiveness. Operants are positively reinforced by A and negatively reinforced by B (i.e., the removal of B reinforces or strengthens the operant).

The aversive A condition is not as clear cut in motivational ramifications. Why, posed Solomon and Corbit [5], would an individual be motivated to engage in contingent operants that are unpleasant and aversive? And, without A, there is no B. As we will see in the case of self-inflicted injury, the anticipated B state is a function of A, such that pain is endured because of a pleasurable after effect. This is a domain that was not foreseen by Solomon and other early opponent process researchers. Nevertheless, Solomon and Corbit discuss social pressures that presage such activities as mountain climbing and parachuting; over time, with repetitions, the punitive A state attenuates, while the positively reinforcing B increases in strength. Over time, the weakened A condition may become a positive reinforcer. And do not forget that conditioned Pavlovian stimuli (e.g., mountain climbing gear; sight of the packaged parachute) may trigger an elevated B condition in the absence of the aversive A.

Recapitulation of OPT, Learning, and Motivation

1. Reinforcers are motivators.
2. If the A process is pleasurable, then the anticipation of the pleasurable emotional change becomes motivational.

3. The derived pleasure motivates repeating the action that produces A.
4. Each time the individual engages in actions producing the A state, the antagonist B state will either be initiated or strengthened.
5. The B condition decays slowly.
6. Neutral stimuli that are present and directly preceding the pleasurable A onset can become conditioned to A and become positive secondary reinforcers.
7. Neutral stimuli that are present following the positive A termination and persist to the peak of B may become classically conditioned to B and will have aversive or pleasurable concomitants.
8. Stimuli conditioned to B; therefore, they become secondary positive or negative reinforcers.
9. Negative reinforcers will energize (i.e., motivate) escape and avoidance behaviors. Remember, negative reinforcers gain power via their removal or absence. Therefore, an adverse B condition or associated secondary negative reinforcers motivate engaging in operants that provide avoidance or escape from anticipated adverse consequences of B.
10. Finally, and axiomatically, in instances where A is aversive (e.g., self-injuries), and endured to produce the B after effect, neutral stimuli will become secondary negative and positive reinforcers, respectively.

References

1. Hilgard ER, Bower GH. Theories of learning. Prentice-Hall; 1975.
2. Longe JL. The gale encyclopedia of psychology. Gale Cengage; 2016.
3. Pavlov IP. Conditioned reflexes and psychiatry. New York: International Publishers; 1941.
4. Hilgard ER, Bower G. Pavlov's classical conditioning theories of learning. Englewood Cliffs: Prentice-Hall; 1975.
5. Solomon RL, Corbit JD. An opponent-process theory of motivation: I. Temporal dynamics of affect. Psychol Rev. 1974;81(2):119–45. Available from: https://doi.org/10.1037/h0036128.

6. Raskin DC. Semantic conditioning and generalization of autonomic responses. J Exp Psychol. 1969;79(1):69–76. Available from: https://doi.org/10.1037/h0026907.
7. Kershaw JC, Running CA. Conditioning of human salivary flow using a visual cue for sour candy. Arch Oral Biol. 2018;92:90–5. Available from: https://doi.org/10.1016/j.archoralbio.2018.05.010.
8. Brotsky SJ. Classical conditioning of the galvanic skin response to verbal concepts. J Exp Psychol. 1968;76(2):244–53. Available from: https://doi.org/10.1037/h0025371.
9. Krypotos A-M, Mertens G, Leer A, Engelhard IM. Induction of conditioned avoidance via mental imagery. Behav Res Ther. 2020;132:103652. Available from: https://doi.org/10.1016/j.brat.2020.103652.
10. Thurber S. Effect size estimates in chemical aversion treatments of alcoholism. J Clin Psychol. 1985;41(2):285–7. Available from: https://doi.org/10.1002/1097-4679(198503)41:23.0.co;2-h.
11. Skinner B. The behavior of organisms: an experimental analysis. Appleton-Century; 1938.
12. Weiss SJ, Rosales-Ruiz J. Operant/classical conditioning: comparisons, intersections and interactions the 2014 winter conference on animal learning and behavior focus and research seminar sessions. Int J Comp Psychol. 2014;27(4):515–25. Available from: https://doi.org/10.46867/ijcp.2014.27.04.07.
13. Mahlberg J, Seabrooke T, Weidemann G, Hogarth L, Mitchell CJ, Moustafa AA. Human appetitive Pavlovian-to-instrumental transfer: a goal-directed account. Psychol Res. 2021;85(2):449–63. Available from: https://doi.org/10.1007/s00426-019-01266-3.
14. Donahoe J. Biological behaviorism. In: Zillo D, editor. Contemporary behaviorisms in debate. Springer Nature; 2021. p. 113–35.
15. Schlund MW, Cataldo MF. Amygdala involvement in human avoidance, escape and approach behavior. NeuroImage. 2010;53(2):769–76. Available from: https://doi.org/10.1016/j.neuroimage.2010.06.058.
16. Sege CT, Bradley MM, Lang PJ. Avoidance and escape: defensive reactivity and trait anxiety. Behav Res Ther. 2018;104:62–8. Available from: https://doi.org/10.1016/j.brat.2018.03.002.
17. Walker C, Hedberg A, Clement P, Wright L. Clinical procedures for behavior therapy. Englewood Cliffs: Prentice-Hall; 1981.
18. Seward JP. Drive, incentive, and reinforcement. Psychol Rev. 1956;63(3):195–203. Available from: https://doi.org/10.1037/h0048229.
19. Cofer C, Appley M. Motivation: theory and research. Wiley; 1964.
20. Heise M, Werthmann J, Murphy F, Tuschen-Caffier B, Renner F. Imagine how good that feels: the impact of anticipated positive emotions on motivation for reward activities. Cogn Ther Res. 2022;46(4):704–20. Available from: https://doi.org/10.1007/s10608-022-10306-z.

Practical Implications

8

Preamble

The data reviewed in the prior chapters suggest that in addition to chemical usage disorders, a variety of other maladaptive behavioral manifestations may adhere to an opponent process model of addiction, viz., a shift in motivation from an initial state of disequilibrium to a compensatory, emotional contrast. As presented, even ostensive altruistic behaviors such as blood donation may fall under the opponent process rubric.

Model and Theory Related to OP

The OPT model is composed of constructs or words with denotative explicitness and their relationships. Basic to OPT are the A and B processes, hedonic contrasts, and acquired motivation. When the constructs of a model are adequately connected to the world of reality (e.g., human physiology and environmental determinants), over time, the model may become a theory, acceptable to members of the scientific community. In brief, a theory can be tested and potentially refuted, a model cannot [1].

The reviewed data suggests OPT may have explanatory power and relevance to certain human disorders and adjustment prob-

J. W. Gibson et al., *Opponent Process Theory*,
https://doi.org/10.1007/978-3-032-00090-3_8

lems as well as germane to more prosaic endeavors and even altruistic actions. Throughout the book, and indeed in the book's title, we have referred to opponent process formulations as "theory"; we aver that such an appellation is not inappropriate; importantly, there is nothing as practical as a good scientific theory.

Application

As mentioned, OPT provides extrapolation of a unique addiction perspective (acquired motivation) both to understanding and treatment of certain human disorders such as and obviously chemical usage problems. The treatment model includes integration with data generated from theories of learning, viz., Pavlov and Skinner. We will illustrate application specific to the treatment of chemical dependency, non-suicidal self-injuries, and eating disorders, areas that have OPT explanations and are of pervasive concern. In this chapter, we will introduce the latest iteration of applied learning theory, evaluative conditioning.

Factors Associated with Effective Therapeutic Interventions

Insight Insight can be defined as "a sudden change in or on the formation of a concept or other type of knowledge representation often leading to the solution of a problem" [2]. Insight into psychotherapy refers to the goal of promoting an understanding and awareness of the cause of current emotional and behavioral difficulties. In some therapeutic techniques, the ultimate goal is insight; in others, insight is viewed as a necessary but not sufficient for therapeutic improvement. Regardless, OPT may provide a comprehensible, scientifically based explanation for disorders that likely are not part of an individual's common sensical speculation, one that engenders "sudden illumination."

Furthermore, the mysterious, difficult to understand nature of certain psychiatric disorders such as non-suicidal self-injuries

(NSSI), chemical addictions, and food-related maladies (and perhaps other mental and emotional dysfunctions) can be unraveled and rendered comprehensible with reference to the fundamental OP principles of hedonic contrast and acquired motivation. The additional neurophysiological and environmental learning components of opponent process theory connect the constructs to palpable reality, perhaps enhancing its appeal and acceptability to patients oriented to a methodological naturalism approach to truth in contrast to therapeutic modalities lacking a scientific foundation.

Congruence An effective therapeutic intervention may require that a patient perceives a congruence between the nature of the presenting problems and the type of therapy implemented. For instance, if a maladaptive behavioral pattern is viewed by the patient as being acquired via learning, a modality based on unlearning or extinction would likely be acceptable to the individual. If a patient perceives congruence between the nature of the problem and the nature of the treatment, therapy becomes more acceptable; with acceptance, it can be posited that the likelihood of compliance to therapy requirements (e.g., "homework" assignments) is increased. And, importantly, if the elements of therapy have verified scientific effectiveness, so much the incentive for adherence to therapeutic requirements. More explicit to OPT, if a patient accedes to the model presented in this text, basically a model of generalized addiction, whether, for example, to chemicals or self-injuries, treatment modalities consistent with the model are likely acceptable and adhered to (see Meichenbaum and Turk [3] for further elucidation).

Motivation and OPT

An effective intervention subsumes a documented change in behavior. Applied OPT then refers to procedures that produce behavioral change, and change requires motivation.

As discussed in the previous chapter, a motive is a spring to action; it involves the activation of behavior. At the most basic level, motives are the "drives" that "push" the individual into action. The classic exemplars are the irritating biological deficits or needs, such as hunger and thirst that actuate and direct behavior toward goals that will reduce the drive state and eliminate the irritating internal instigator (i.e., access to food and water). Drive states such as thirst "push" the organism into action while enhancing the stimulus value of events associated with need satisfaction (e.g., supermarkets with access to food and drinking fountains). Although not necessary for survival, a strong, aversive B condition in OPT can be viewed as an acquired drive or "push" motive, leading to actions geared to reducing the irritant or facilitating a return to homeostasis.

Drive states are ubiquitous for living organisms. In addition to biological drives, human motives can involve more complicated mental processes. Perhaps the best single definition of motivation at the human level, one that is readily incorporated into opponent process theory, is the following: *anticipation of affective change*. Anticipation of a future event is a cognitive process. Affective is the term used by psychologists for emotion. If one anticipates that a particular behavior will lead to a positive emotional change, this will arouse and energize engagement in that behavior. If the individual anticipates that a behavior will lead to a negative emotional change, there is arousal related to avoiding this behavioral act. These are the future anticipated conditions that "pull" the individual into activity [4].

Specifics of OPT Motivation

When A Is Positive

The A condition can be pleasurable or aversive; both emotional states have somewhat different motivational dynamics. The positive A condition adheres to our definition of motivation above, "the anticipation of a positive change in affect" that impels and energizes action. The B state, or hedonic contrast, constitutes an irritant that pushes or drives the individual in directions that will provide reduction or escape from the aversiveness. Operants for A are positive reinforcers; operants for B are negative reinforcers. And reinforcers motivate approach, avoidance, and escape behaviors.

When A Is Adverse

The attractive, motivational valence of a positive A state accounts for the initial activation of behavior. The aversive A condition is not as clear cut in motivational ramifications. Why, posed Solomon and Corbit [4], would an individual be motivated to engage in contingent operants that are unpleasant and aversive? And, without A, there is no B. As we will see in the case of self-inflicted injury, the anticipated B state is a function of A, such that pain in endured because of a pleasurable after effect. This is a domain that was not foreseen by Solomon and other early opponent process researchers. Nevertheless, Solomon and Corbit discuss social pressures that presage such activities as mountain climbing, and parachuting; over time, with repetitions, the punitive A state attenuates while the positively reinforcing B increases in strength. Over time, the weakened A condition may become a positive reinforcer. And remember that conditioned Pavlovian stimuli (e.g., mountain climbing gear; sight of the packaged parachute) may trigger an elevated B condition in the absence of the aversive A.

Treatment Modalities

Stimulus Control and Habit Strength

Effective OPT interventions are intertwined with two related learning principles instilled from the theories of Pavlov and Skinner: Stimulus control and habit strength.

These are notions that have been mainstream in the behavioral therapy literature for decades. They represent rather extreme positions on the effects of environmental conditions and behavior.

Perhaps this is best represented by the statement, "the best predictor of a person's current behavior is the environmental setting in which she/he resides or interacts." If a student is in the college library, there is an elevated probability that she/he is engaged in some type of scholarly activity. Stimuli in the library (books, tables, other students engaged in study) exert "power" over actions via classical conditioning and as the student behaves in conformance to implied or direct rules of library deportment, behavioral habits or "habit strength" increases via Skinnerian principles elaborated by Clark Hull [5].

Again, a stimulus is anything that activates a sensory organ. Stimuli can be internal, within the individual, or external (environmental) in nature. Environmental stimuli exert control over one's behavior via Pavlovian conditioning. As discussed, Pavlovian conditioning pertains to the autonomic nervous system and relates to stimuli-emotionality learning. Whatever the initial source of an emotional reaction is, neutral environmental stimuli may acquire "*stimulus control*," via temporal/spatial contiguity. Again, regarding OP, stimuli that directly evoke the A condition (e.g., affective impact of alcohol ingestion and nicotine from cigarette smoking) and neutral stimuli that become contiguously conditioned to the A affective state (sight of alcohol containers; taste of alcoholic beverage; cigarette cartons in grocery stores) together with neutral stimuli contiguously conditioned to the B state, after the ascendency in strength of the B state (i.e., addiction), formerly neutral stimuli that become conditioned stimuli may act as eliciting stimuli. It is also possible for multiple stimuli to become classically conditioned to the hedonic contrast. This in part is what is meant by stimulus control, from the OP perspective. When the B state is adverse, the conditioned stimuli may evoke craving, or drive motivation, together with motivation to avoid or escape the craving. Of course, in the case of chemical addiction, one way to avoid or escape is a return to drug usage.

Practical Ramifications

1. *Become aware of situations that trigger maladaptive A or B conditions* and avoid placing yourself in proximity such situational cues.
2. Conversely, place yourself in situations devoid of such eliciting cues.
3. If cues are "internalized" in internal dialogues (self-talk) and mental imagery, procedures for thought modification and thought stopping can be employed.
4. Paradoxically, consider exposing and indeed satiating yourself to maladaptive while resisting escape tendencies; over time, the cues may habituate or extinguish, loosing eliciting power.

Introduction to Evaluative Conditioning

Opponent process theory is a form of acquired motivation, with the shift in affect being a major component thereof. Whereas this emotional change is the result of physiological homeostatic mechanisms in OPT, the emotional change instigated in evaluative conditioning (EC) is via direct contiguous association. EC (or TEC) simply focuses on the affective valence of a disordered behavior and targets an affective valence change through Pavlovian conditioning. More specifically, ECT involves repeated paring of an unconditioned stimulus (e.g., an aversive visual stimulus such as a picture of a cockroach) that elicits an automatic emotional reaction that becomes attached to stimulus material having an ostensive positive valence (e.g., a pornographic image, for an individual with the desire to overcome an apparent addiction to pornography). The resultant association is between the CS and in this example an object with unpleasant valence [6, 7]. The goal is to attain a shift in valence of the pornographic material and a possible acquired motivational behavioral change (e.g., from approach to avoidance or escape). In the scientific literature on this topic, there are two subcategories of evaluative conditioning: “Therapeutic Evaluative Conditioning” and “Cue Exposure” (see Hofmann et al. [8], for a meta-analysis and additional information on evaluative conditioning).

Evaluative Conditioning and Aversive Conditioning

In *Aversive Evaluative Conditioning*, for example, a hospitalized patient diagnosed with “alcohol usage disorder” is administered emetine, a chemical that induces nausea and vomiting. As the patient begins to experience the aversive effects of emetine, she/he is taken to a treatment room in which the patient’s favorite alcoholic beverage is poured into a large glass. The patient begins with olfactory stimulation, smelling the beverage. As the nausea continues to increase in intensity, the patient then tastes beverage followed by ingesting copious amounts. This is followed by regurgitation into a container while remaining in close proximity to smell the emesis. This is repeated several times on alternate days for 2 weeks. The typical result is that the smell and taste of the beverage evokes nausea, in the absence of the emetine. Importantly, smell and taste of the alcoholic beverage become conditioned stimuli in “aversion therapy” and elicit a response, nausea, incompatible with alcohol ingestion [9, 10]. It is noteworthy that although this form of treatment is very effective for alcoholism, it is also difficult for a patient to undergo procedures that result in nausea and vomiting; persons with alcohol use disorder are likely to seek treatment options that are easier to endure [10]. Furthermore, aversive conditioning requires hospitalization and medical supervision. To our knowledge, there are no longer any emetine-related treatment programs remaining in the United States; Schick Shadel, the last hospital to offer such aversive therapy treatment, ceased operations in 2023.

Evaluative Conditioning for Alcohol Addiction

Aversive conditioning and evaluative conditioning (EC) for alcohol use disorder share the same goal, reducing or eliminating alcohol ingestion. EC approaches involve comparatively mild noxious stimuli and require much less time to implement in contrast to emetics. For instance, Tello et al. [11] exposed problem drinkers to a computer-assisted task that required only 5 min to administer. Words related to alcohol usage were paired with negative pictures, whereas words related to soft drink ingestion were paired with positive pictures. This brief EC intervention reduced drinking behavior significantly in comparison to a non-intervention control group.

Evaluative Conditioning and Other Chemical Usage Disorders

Remember that any neutral stimulus (neutral meaning that it lacks any initial power to evoke an autonomic nervous system response; stimulus meaning anything that activates a sensory organ) can be associated in time (contiguously) with A and B states and thus gain Pavlovian power to evoke those states in the future. Now try to imagine the kinds of stimuli that might be present to potentially become respondents and secondary operants. For "A" conditioned stimuli, we have (depending on the type of drug ingested) (1) a syringe, (2) shot glass, (3) kitchen utensils, etc. For the B condition, imagine neutral stimuli that might be present during times of forced drug abstinence or volitional attempts to abstain from chemical usage: Stimuli extant in incarceration, lack of money, persons in alcoholic or narcotic anonymous groups, members of a church congregation, etc.

Second, the goal for most individuals who desire to overcome an addition is complete abstinence from the chemical in question, albeit in the domain of alcoholism the debate over complete abstinence versus controlled drinking is still extant [12]. From the OPT perspective, if the intervals between alcohol ingestion periods are sufficiently distributed over time, the opponent process is unlikely to perpetuate to the point of addiction. This perspective is supported in a recent Meta-analytic review [13].

Principles from opponent process theory and related operant and Pavlovian learning offer both an understanding of the nature of addiction and knowledge about factors that influence relapse (e.g., conditioned environmental stimuli). Of primary importance are that laws that govern the process of addiction can also be used to reduce the probability of returning to chemical usage during a period of abstinence.

Cue Exposure: Nicotine Addiction (Cravings)

Nicotine addiction cravings reflect classical conditioning of an opponent process.

Pavlovian Conditioning

1. UCS (ingestion of nicotine via smoking) → NS (ashtray) → UCR (affect elevation via dopamine)
2. CS (ashtray) → CR (affect elevation)
3. Conditioned response opponent process (negative affect such as anxiety)
4. CS (ashtray) → CR (hedonic contrast, anxiety)

   A conditioned cue now evokes a negative opponent process (anxiety) producing motivation to escape the anxiety via return to nicotine ingestion, i.e., craving for the UCS.

Cue Exposure Therapy combines Pavlovian extinction interventions with evaluative Conditioning [14].

Unrod et al. [14] exposed cigarette smoking volunteers to Images (visual cues) that evoke cravings on computer screens across twice weekly sessions for 6 weeks. The stimuli included pictures of people, situations, places, and other things commonly associated with nicotine cravings, or what we have deemed the B opponent process. The program was unique in tailoring the procedures to the individual participants. That is, the participants also provided their own photographs of stimuli personally found to elicit cravings. Moreover, the intervention included in vivo psychomotor experiences such as handling and smelling of cigarettes, ashtrays, and lighters. This was a Pavlovian extinction procedure, exposing the individual to conditioned cues in the absence of the UCS, the actual nicotine from cigarette smoking.

The aversive EC method involved pairing the smoking and craving cues with negative affect images, pictures depicting sad and anxious human facial expressions. Resultant measures of nicotine craving were significantly reduced by the end of the brief implemented treatment.

Therapeutic Evaluative Conditioning (TEC) for Self-injurious Behavior (SIB)

TEC is an alternate phrase for or subcategory of evaluative conditioning applied to a mood elevation B process, explicitly to the motivational hedonic contrast engendered by self-inflicted injury.

Pavlovian Aversive conditioning involves stimuli that promote rather extreme autonomic nervous system reactions (e.g., nausea; shock-related pain); in contrast, TEC is an attenuated aversive subtype with the goal of motivating behavioral change by engendering a valence shift from pleasant to unpleasant.

As elaborated in Chap. 6, self-inflicted pain (e.g., cutting; burning) can arouse a euphoric B contrast that motivates repeated self-injuries. Visual images such as the sight of cutaneous injuries can become conditioned to the positive B state and develop eliciting properties. In TEC, mildly noxious stimuli are contiguously associated with these conditioned visual images.

Researchers in the Mathew Nock laboratory at Harvard University concocted a mobile device to facilitate TEC for individuals who engage in self-injuries. Although the causes of self-harm are likely multifarious, an OPT interpretation is certainly tenable, and TEC can be viewed as logically consonant with OPT principles (hence, there is a potential facilitation of therapeutic effectiveness through insight via congruence with and understanding of the OPT model).

TEC was adapted into a memory game using a mobile appliance in which points are earned for remembering and identifying associated stimuli as rapidly as possible. The stimuli can be written words (e.g., "dangerous") and photographs. Embedded among the stimuli are pictures of cutaneous burns, cuts, or other forms physical injuries. In the precursor to the game, pairs of stimuli are presented that require memorization. In simplified form, one pair might be a photograph of a cutaneous cut and a picture of a burned area of the skin. Another pair might be photos of a spider and a snake or the words "death," and "dangerous," as well as positive and neutral pairings. After memorizing the initial paired stimuli, the "memory" game commences. The participant, an individual with a history of SIB, is then presented a series of stimuli and is required to identify correctly the previously memorized pairings. The participant is unaware that regardless of correctness, the injurious stimuli are being contiguously conditioned to the observed noxious stimuli. The game becomes more complicated in a stage progression with an increasing number of presented stimuli. It also repeatedly returns to new memorization of stimulus pairs and an iteration of the aforementioned procedures. In three independent studies of TEC for individuals with a history of self-injurious behaviors, a conditioned emotional aversion to NSSI was demonstrated together with attendant reductions in self-injuries [15, 16]. More specific details about this research are given below.

As observed in Image 8.1, TEC is initiated with three sets of paired stimuli to be memorized (upper left corner). Included is a pairing of two types of cutaneous injuries, one of a cut, the other scraped skin. In the figure, the game begins (lower left corner) with a 2 × 2 presentation that includes the memorized cutaneous injury pairings to be identified for winning points. The participant is required to select as rapidly as possible the two associated injury images. While so doing, there will be a fortuitous Pavlovian association of the cutaneous injuries with the word "danger" and a possibly aversive picture of a spider. The therapeutic game continues with repetitive associations of aversive stimuli and a variety of SIB images, with progressive levels of difficulty. Following a

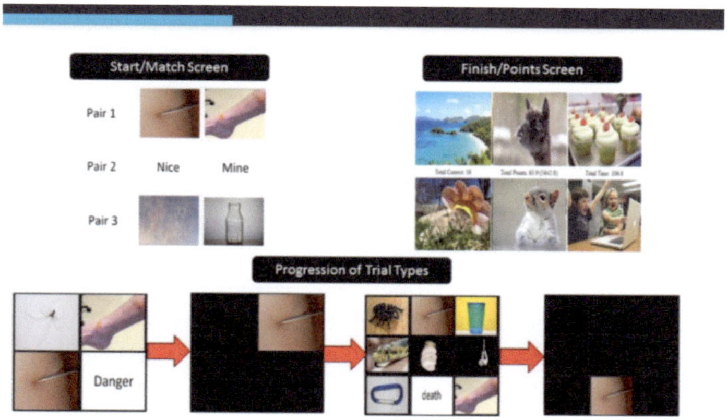

Image 8.1 Therapeutic evaluative conditioning. (Copyrighted figure. Permission from John Wiley & Sons)

series of 2 × 2 presentations, for instance, there is a shift within the game. Now when the individual selects the single cutaneous cut image, the other 2 × 2 images are masked (lower center) and immediately a more complicated 3 × 3 grid appears (third from the lower left). This 3 × 3 grid contains the designated SIB pairings along with the word "death," a new arachnoid image, and four other pictured stimuli, requiring greater attentional vigilance in the context of time pressure.

It is again important to note that the TEC approach was implemented without the awareness by the self-injurious participants and it still demonstrated effectiveness. Nevertheless, there is evidence that increased efficacy obtains when TEC participants are informed about the purpose and rationale of TEC [8]; further, this awareness would potentially enhance treatment via the congruence principle (above). In addition, we have focused on the aversive elements of TEC consistent with the goal of reducing the positive valance of the B process. TEC can also be employed to augment more favorable self-perceptions, often a part of the issue both in SIB and eating disorders [8]. Finally, it is noteworthy that the impact of TEC may fade over time [15]. This is an expected extinction phenomenon in any type of Pavlovian conditioning.

Enhanced awareness of TEC principles combined with periodic "reinforcement" treatments are likely required for longer term maintenance.

Note Procedures like TEC can be self-administered through mental imagery. If, for example, you desire to expunge or attenuate ingesting chocolate candy, repeatedly imagine a piece of the candy on your kitchen table right next to several dead cockroaches. In a procedure termed "covert sensitization," the individual records a complete story replete with aversive consequences associated with the sight or ingestion of chocolate candy and periodically listens to the recording.

Eating Disorders

We have discussed two topics that constitute DSM disorders, viz., chemical usage and SIB, also termed non-suicidal self-injuries (NSSI). A third topic, eating disorders, was only mentioned in an earlier chapter on the dopaminergic and neurophysiological aspects of food ingestion, with the promise of further explication of eating abnormalities in this, the application chapter.

Chemical addiction and SIB are clearly relevant to opponent process theory as an explanatory construct. In the food/eating section, we introduced some additional neurophysiological components that will now be discussed in greater detail.

The ingestion of food has a demonstrable dopaminergic effect and likely engenders a counter reaction or what we have termed the hedonic contrast, or B state called "hunger." This is consistent with the opponent process formulation. We have also posited that for individuals with propensities toward eating disorders, there exist characteristics that augment this counter-reaction or B process, rendering it stronger and perhaps increasing its rate of progression. Persons with such predispositions have an elevated level of trait anxiety and distorted thoughts pertaining to body image and weight gain. Such specific person characteristics need to be incorporated into the opponent process equation to account for eating disorders. Furthermore, these pre-existing traits lead to a disruption of the physiological aspects of opponent process theory.

Neurophysiology of Eating Disorders

Consistent with information presented on the biological Underpinnings of OPT (Chap. 2), the ventral striatum (VS) is an important brain structure in opponent process theory albeit we have emphasized one subcomponent thereof, the so-called pleasure center or nucleus accumbens (NAc). The VS itself is regarded as an important motor activation structure of the brain. In "normal" eating behavior, the hypothalamus is the structure that initiates the "starting" (Lateral region) and "stopping" (Ventral Medial region) of eating by signaling for motor activity mediated by the VS (see Image 8.2) Specifically, in addition to its importance in reward circuity, the NAc actuates behaviors pertaining to searching for and finding rewarding activities (such as favorable foods) as well as avoiding outcomes that may be non-rewarding or aversive. The other VS division is termed "Tubular Striatum" (TuS) that facilitates actual consummatory actions (e.g., food ingestion). Another way of putting it, the NAc is active in "seeking," the TuS in "taking" [17].

In the eating disorder literature, the VS is often noted as important in actuating motor behavior although noteworthy is not distinguishing the disparate functions of the two divisions.

Importantly, the regions of the VS can be influenced by the individual's ruminations about body image, fear of weight gain, and maintenance of "thinness." Seidel et al. [18] reported functional MRI data indicating negative self-talk by eating disorder patients affected neural regulation of eating behavior via the ventral striatum. Moreover, ecological monitoring assessments supported the notion that such maladaptive thinking extended into real life situations producing negative affect and eating disorder symptomatology.

The components of the VS are part of the Hypothalamus → Ventral Striatum circuitry that is ascendant in the regulation of

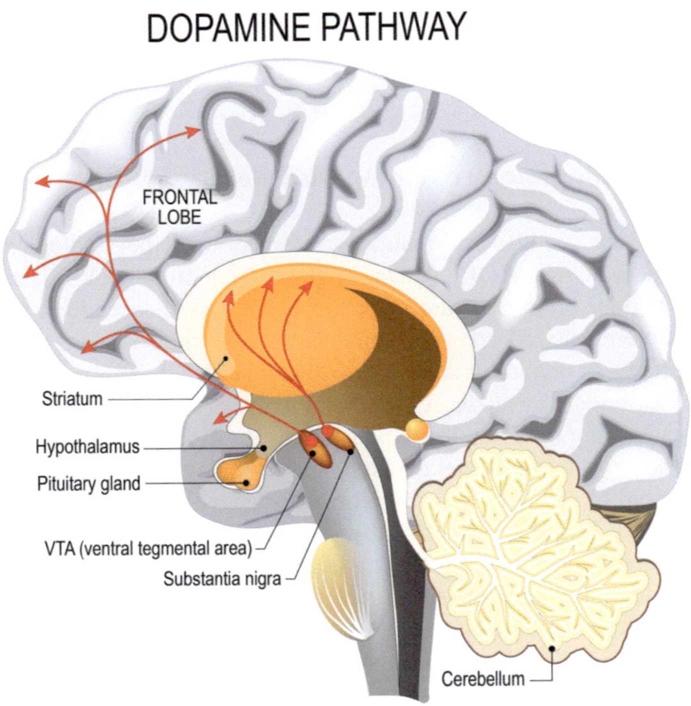

Image 8.2 Dopamine pathway. (Usage Rights Granted by IStock)

hunger and eating behavior. In normal eating, the direction of effective dopaminergic connectivity in this circuity is from the hypothalamus to the VS. One region of the Hypothalamus (lateral) signals the VS (NAc and TuS) to start the motor activity involved in food ingestion; the other region (ventral medial) signals the VS to terminate eating behavior. This "normal" circuity involves dopamine as the neurotransmitter.

At the neurophysiologic level, there is a reversal of directionality between the hypothalamus and ventral striatum. In "normal" eating, the starting and stopping is regulated by the hypothalamus through the motor activity engendered by the regions of the ventral striatum. In eating disorders, the normal pathway is compromised in what Frank et al. [19] term a "fear-driven dopamine-mediated circuitry" in which the directionality is reversed, from the ventral striatum to the hypothalamus. Now hunger cues (part of the B process) are either overridden as in anorexia or poorly regulated, as in bulimia.

Extrapolating from the current literature, we aver that food ingestion is dopaminergic and tentatively postulate congruence with opponent process dynamics. Hunger and related emotionality may be a manifestation of a "B" process. It can further be posited that an individual with propensities toward an eating disorder may have elevated trait anxiety that increases the intensity of the hedonic contrasting "B" state. Moreover, the B state among persons with eating disorders will likely be augmented by ruminations about body image and thinness. Conditioned extrinsic cues as well as internal semantic stimuli (i.e., maladaptive self-speech; semantic aversive conditioning) will further combine, increase, and trigger the B condition in the absence of eating behavior. Even very sporadic eating will strengthen an unusually elevated B state in eating disorders, one more difficult to extinguish than would otherwise be the case. Eventually, the survival motivation pertaining to food ingestion is regulated by the opposing B process. This also suggests the behavioral treatments espoused in this chapter, consistent with OPT, may also apply to eating disorders.

TEC employed by Franklin et al. [15] were previously discussed with emphasis on changing the aftermath of self-inflicted pain from pleasant to unpleasant. Their work also includes EC directed toward producing more positive emotionality in the individual's self-perception via presentation of pleasant words and visual stimuli contiguously with the word "self."

Evaluative Conditioning and Eating Disorders

Aspen et al. [20] implemented EC procedures to change adverse emotionality related to bodily dissatisfaction. Eligible participants were women who based on pre-study assessment were deemed at high risk for developing eating disorders, with elevated body dissatisfaction and expressed eating concerns. Selected participants changed to standard fitted clothing and submitted to three full body photographs (front, left, and right profiles). They were then randomly assigned to treatment and control (waitlist) conditions.

One of the three pictures of a treatment participant's body was presented at random in one of four quadrants on a computer screen. The remaining three quadrants contained pictures of other women's bodies. The participant was instructed to click on each of the four pictures as rapidly as possible. With each selected quadrant, a new picture appeared. This was replicated in 270 trials over a 3- to 5-min time period and repeated for three subsequent weeks. The evaluative conditioning aspect was that the replacement picture for the self-photo was always a smiling face; replacement pictures for the other women's bodies were either neutral in facial features or frowning. The short-term results indicated significant declines in concerns for weight and body shape together with increased self-esteem levels; the improvements in bodily dissatisfaction were maintained over a 12-week period. Moreover, in a rather novel research approach, the evaluative conditioning procedures were later implemented with the control sample producing similar positive findings.

In sum, eating disorders appear to fit an opponent process model with hunger being either overcontrolled or intermittently and sporadically controlled by a B process. Moreover, the opponent B process may be intensified by ruminations concerning adverse bodily appearance. It appears that weight and body dissatisfactions can potentially be modified by evaluative conditioning, thus reducing B intensity. A therapeutic supplement, if needed, pertains to thought analysis and thought-stopping techniques (below).

Thought Analysis and Thought Stopping

If negative body-related thoughts adversely affect the neurophysiology of eating behavior, procedures designed to improve feelings about oneself through evaluative conditioning are reasonable interventions. Techniques for reducing or eliminating such thinking directly can also be used singly or in combination with EC. Although there are a variety of thought-stopping modalities, we advocate the following:

Thought Analysis

As a precursor to eliminating or attenuating an unwanted thought, it is important to make an informed decision; some personally irritating or harmful thoughts may nonetheless need to remain in conscious awareness for discussion with a confidant or mental health professional. Engagement in the procedures below are recommended for delineation of a thought or thoughts that should be expunged:

1. Since we tend to think in words, consider thought to be covert self-speech or internal monologues.
2. Select the internal monologue that pertains to words you say to yourself about your weight and body image.
3. Write down the thought.
4. Rate your degree of belief in the thought. Do you really believe the self-talk or is it some type of exaggeration or distortion?
5. Count and record the number of times in a given time period that you are aware of covert rehearsal (frequency) of the thought.
6. Consider the advantages and disadvantages of continuing to engage in the thought.
7. Decision-(a) continue the thought; (b) reduce the thought; (c) eliminate the thought.
8. If the decision is to reduce or expunge the thought, try thought stopping.

Thought Stopping [21, 22]

1. Continue to monitor the frequency of the thought.
2. Associate mild pain every time the thought occurs-hold your breath; pinch yourself; "zap" yourself with a rubber band around your wrist.
3. If you are alone, say out loud, assertively = Stop! Stop! Stop!
4. Creatively generate and use "coping" phrases, alternate thoughts you really believe that can be substituted for the word or phrase you are trying to attenuate or eliminate. For instance, rather than ruminating on what you have determined to be a

maladaptive series of body-related verbalizations, substitute, "this thought is harmful"; "this thought is causing eating problem"; "this thought is not valid." Again, any coping thought requires veridicality, pertaining to elements that are acceptable and believed, based on evidence.

References

1. Passey D. Theories, theoretical and conceptual frameworks, models and constructs: limiting research outcomes through misconceptions and misunderstandings. 2020. Available from: https://doi.org/10.21428/8c225f6e.56810a1a.
2. Kounios J. The cognitive neuroscience of insight. Front Hum Neurosci. 2018;12. Available from: https://doi.org/10.3389/conf.fnhum.2018.227.00132.
3. Meichenbaum D, Turk D. Facilitating treatment adherence: a practitioner's guide. Springer; 1987.
4. Solomon RL, Corbit JD. An opponent-process theory of motivation: I. Temporal dynamics of affect. Psychol Rev. 1974;81(2):119–45. Available from: https://doi.org/10.1037/h0036128.
5. Hilgard E, Bower G. Theories of learning. Englewood Cliffs: Prentice-Hall; 1975.
6. Sweldens S, Van Osselaer SMJ, Janiszewski C. Evaluative conditioning procedures and the resilience of conditioned brand attitudes. J Consum Res. 2010;37(3):473–89. Available from: https://doi.org/10.1086/653656.
7. Moran T, Nudler Y, Bar-Anan Y. Evaluative conditioning: past, present, and future. Annu Rev Psychol. 2023;74(1):245–69. Available from: https://doi.org/10.1146/annurev-psych-032420-031815.
8. Hofmann W, De Houwer J, Perugini M, Baeyens F, Crombez G. Evaluative conditioning in humans: a meta-analysis. Psychol Bull. 2010;136(3):390–421. Available from: https://doi.org/10.1037/a0018916.
9. Thurber S. Effect size estimates in chemical aversion treatments of alcoholism. J Clin Psychol. 1985;41(2):285–7. Available from: https://doi.org/10.1002/1097-4679(198503)41:23.0.co;2-h.
10. Wiens AN, Menustik CE. Treatment outcome and patient characteristics in an aversion therapy program for alcoholism. Am Psychol. 1983;38(10):1089–96. Available from: https://doi.org/10.1037/0003-066x.38.10.1089.
11. Tello N, Bocage-Barthélémy Y, Dandaba M, Jaafari N, Chatard A. Evaluative conditioning: a brief computer-delivered intervention to

reduce college student drinking. Addict Behav. 2018;82:14–8. Available from: https://doi.org/10.1016/j.addbeh.2018.02.018.
12. Eddie D, Bergman BG, Hoffman LA, Kelly JF. Abstinence versus moderation recovery pathways following resolution of a substance use problem: prevalence, predictors, and relationship to psychosocial well-being in a U.S. national sample. Alcohol Clin Exp Res. 2022;46(2):312–25. Available from: https://doi.org/10.1111/acer.14765.
13. Henssler J, Müller M, Carreira H, Bschor T, Heinz A, Baethge C. Controlled drinking—non-abstinent versus abstinent treatment goals in alcohol use disorder: a systematic review, meta-analysis and meta-regression. Addiction. 2021;116(8):1973–87. Available from: https://doi.org/10.1111/add.15329.
14. Unrod M, Drobes DJ, Stasiewicz PR, Ditre JW, Heckman B, Miller RR, et al. Decline in cue-provoked craving during cue exposure therapy for smoking cessation. Nicotine Tob Res. 2014;16(3):306–15. Available from: https://doi.org/10.1093/ntr/ntt145.
15. Franklin JC, Fox KR, Franklin CR, Kleiman EM, Ribeiro JD, Jaroszewski AC, et al. A brief mobile app reduces nonsuicidal and suicidal self-injury: evidence from three randomized controlled trials. J Consult Clin Psychol. 2016;84(6):544–57. Available from: https://doi.org/10.1037/ccp0000093.
16. Franklin JC, Fox KR, Ribeiro JD. How to implement therapeutic evaluative conditioning in a clinical setting. J Clin Psychol. 2017;73(5):559–69. Available from: https://doi.org/10.1002/jclp.22453.
17. Wright KN, Wesson DW. The tubular striatum and nucleus accumbens distinctly represent reward-taking and reward-seeking. J Neurophysiol. 2021;125(1):166–83. Available from: https://doi.org/10.1152/jn.00495.2020.
18. Seidel M, King JA, Ritschel F, Boehm I, Geisler D, Bernardoni F, et al. Processing and regulation of negative emotions in anorexia nervosa: an fMRI study. Neuroimage Clin. 2018;18:1–8. Available from: https://doi.org/10.1016/j.nicl.2017.12.035.
19. Frank GKW, Shott ME, DeGuzman MC. The neurobiology of eating disorders. Child Adolesc Psychiatr Clin N Am. 2019;28(4):629–40. Available from: https://doi.org/10.1016/j.chc.2019.05.007.
20. Aspen V, Martijn C, Alleva JM, Nagel J, Perret C, Purvis C, et al. Decreasing body dissatisfaction using a brief conditioning intervention. Behav Res Ther. 2015;69:93–9. Available from: https://doi.org/10.1016/j.brat.2015.04.003.
21. Hardy J, Oliver E. Self-talk, positive thinking, and thought stopping. In: Eklund R, editor. Encyclopedia of sport and exercise psychology. Sage; 2014.
22. Bakker GM. In defense of thought stopping. Clin Psychol. 2009;13(2):59–68. Available from: https://doi.org/10.1080/13284200902810452.

9 Epilogue

We began this book with the historical precursors of current opponent process theory. We presented an epistemic foundation for OPT beginning with adversarial notions in philosophy and religion and progressing to greater scientific rigor, particularly the opponent visual afterimages and data from neurophysiological research. Within these prevailing influences emerged the contributions of Soloman and Corbit extending opponent process conceptions to human holistic behavior. And we cannot neglect the inspiration of the documented emotional contrasts evinced by paratroopers before and after parachute jumps. All of this eventually produced refutable hypotheses and a testable model of opponent processes and acquired motivation, constituting the data basis for this book.

In our chapters, we have reviewed published studies testing opponent process principles across several diverse subject matter topics. Some domains have substantial research support (e.g., chemical addiction), while others have promising but less than abundant supporting data (e.g., acupuncture). In addition, we have presented instances in which OPT requires modification or better put, an integration with other neurophysiological systems, as in eating disorders. Nevertheless, we would aver that in the aggregate the foundational postulates of OPT have evidential corroboration. Furthermore, OPT potentially fosters understanding of certain heretofore mysterious maladies and, in combination with

J. W. Gibson et al., *Opponent Process Theory*,
https://doi.org/10.1007/978-3-032-00090-3_9

associative learning principles, provides effective treatment modalities. Yet, we hasten to add that like all scientific theories, the constructs of OPT require continued critical scrutiny, and more work is necessitated regarding replication and extension of OPT principles.

Although we have demonstrated extrapolation of OPT to a fairly wide range of phenomena, we foresee additional applicability in any domain of behavior that pertains to heightened emotionality. The bipolar psychiatric disorder, involving varying degrees of elation and depressive fluctuations, might be one area for future investigation. Another realm of interest relates to erratic athletic performance in which the emotional "high" of success is followed by a juxtaposed opponent "low" or the reverse, of course, and how hedonic contrasts affect subsequent athletic performance. And there are likely many other extensions of OPT awaiting creative researchers.

Index

J. W. Gibson et al., *Opponent Process Theory*,
https://doi.org/10.1007/978-3-032-00090-3

H

I

J

L

M

N

O

MIX
Papier aus verantwortungsvollen Quellen
Paper from responsible sources
FSC® C105338

If you have any concerns about our products,
you can contact us on
ProductSafety@springernature.com

In case Publisher is established outside the EU,
the EU authorized representative is:
Springer Nature Customer Service Center GmbH
Europaplatz 3, 69115 Heidelberg, Germany

Printed by Libri Plureos GmbH
in Hamburg, Germany